My End of the Leash

by Holly Cook

Dedication

For all pet care professionals, especially pet sitters,
who dedicate their lives to caring for pets.

May you never forget the wonder of the love of a pet.

Table of Contents

My life has always been graced with the presence of animals.   My love and compassion for them began at an early age and is what made me an outstanding pet sitter and dog walker.   During my journey, I've experienced much joy and much grief. The grief grew with each new trauma experienced until finally I was left with no compassion. I had lost my sparkle. With work and introspection, my compassion has returned and my life is full of joy. You may be traveling this journey or at least recognize yourself as you read about my story into and recovery from compassion fatigue. My hope is that it will help you.

Furry Friends

I vividly recall sitting on the top step of a white concrete front porch my little bare feet firmly planted on the step below attempting to eat an ice cream cone before it melted in the summer heat.   Next to me sat my best friend, Rusty. I was four years old. He was a perfect specimen of a dog—a steadfast, hearty German Shepherd.

Rusty was tall, but solid, and ran like the wind. His ears were perfect for listening to the whispered secrets of a little girl; secrets that were safe with a dog. His paws were bigger than my hands, which made them perfect for holding. And, his fur was soft and dark and I could bury my face in it when I was sad.

Rusty was the best friend a 4-year-old girl could ever ask for. I was happy that day as he sat next to me. I put my sticky little arm around his shoulders and laid my head on his chest. "Har. Har. Har.", he panted. I felt such love for him in that moment, I dropped my ice cream, put both arms around his rough neck and squeezed as hard as my little arms would squeeze. And that handsome, steadfast, dog bit me in the face. As soon as he had made contact, he recoiled and ran away. I put my hand to my face and began to sob. I instinctively knew it was my fault. I had squeezed him too hard. He was warning me that I was hurting him.

Rusty had held back on the bite. He got in trouble for biting me, but I knew I was the one who should have been punished. Instead, I got a couple of stitches and a lot of extra attention for a few days. Still, the guilt and shame of knowing that I had instigated my best friend to bite my face were a bit overwhelming and more than my four-year-old brain could handle. My parents didn't punish me, so I grounded myself. I didn't completely understand why, but I knew I deserved it. I had learned a valuable lesson about a dog that I loved with my whole heart and I never tried to hug him that hard again. I have no idea what my Dad did to him, and, bless his heart, my Dad never told me.

Later that summer, my big brother and I were running around the backyard with sparklers at twilight. It was hard to see with only a sparkler to light my way. I swung it in the air, making circles and dots and dashes, spinning and singing and running with joy. I didn't see Rusty in the dirt and I tripped over his haunches. The rest of his body was buried in a crater he was enthusiastically digging. I could tell he was digging that hole with as much joy as I had experienced running with the sparkler. I laughed until my insides hurt. My sparkler went out and Rusty popped his head out of the enormous hole he had just dug.

It was then that I saw what looked like a tiny little hand sticking out of his mouth. I shrieked and my Dad came running over.

"What the hell is the matter with you?" he asked.

I was already bawling when I tried to explain that Rusty's stomach hand had come up out of his mouth and I was sure he was going to die. My Dad looked at me like I was delusional and said, "What is a stomach hand?"

I said "Dad, it's the hand that comes up from the stomach to take the food from the mouth and put it in the stomach. Rusty's is hanging out of his mouth. He's going to die!" My sobbing erupted anew.

My Dad just smiled at me. He never said a word. He opened Rusty's mouth very slowly and carefully. I held my breath and watched to see how my Dad was going to put Rusty's stomach hand back into his stomach. I was expecting him to put his hand down a German Shepherd's throat—a German Shepherd that had recently bit me! But, I had confidence in my Dad's ability to be Dad. When he grabbed the stomach hand, I let out a little yelp and he looked at me. I put my hands over my mouth, so I wouldn't make any more noise and my Dad started to PULL the Stomach Hand out of Rusty's mouth! He was sure to die now and I fell into a puddle of tantrumming grief. Why would he pull out the stomach hand? How would Rusty get food? I sobbed and sobbed, inconsolable.

My mom came around the corner wondering what I was carrying on about. I sat up ready to tell what my Dad had done to my dog. Instead, my Dad told her the story. I sat on the grass with tears drying on my face, hoping my mom would tell him to put the stomach hand back where it belonged so Rusty wouldn't die. Instead, she started laughing. I was devastated and felt betrayed by both my parents.

My mom scooped me up in her arms, brushed the hair out of my eyes as she wiped my tears and said,

"Look at what your Dad has". It turned out that Rusty's "stomach hand" was a regular old, ugly mole that Rusty had dug out of the ground and on which he was happily chomping.

I will never forget the feeling that my dog was going to die that day. Even at four years old, I was already tuned into my dog. Fortunately, Rusty was just fine, but the seeds of compassion and empathy towards animals had been planted, and would continue to grow and flourish throughout my life.

To this day, my Dad loves to tell the story about Rusty's stomach hand. The story gets a little more embellished with time and he tends to leave out the part about the sparklers at the beginning. However, he does remember that we continued to play with the sparklers deep into the night until I collided with a tree and hit my head. He likes to tell that part, too.

Rusty wasn't my only loyal companion and friend as a child. We always had pets in our house. Mom loved to garden and we had many dogs named after flowers—Pansy, Petunia, Tulip, just to name a few.

When I was five, my mom got herself a little lap dog and named her Pansy. Pansy was a small Cockapoo dog with brown curly fur, kind eyes, and no tail. When she was happy, her whole body wiggled. Good hearted and fun, she was always up for a game of hide and seek with me in the basement. I had a lot of time to play with her by myself. I only went to school for half a day while my big brother was gone until 4 o'clock.

Pansy and I got to be very good friends and we spent many hours in the basement. I can't recall if she wasn't allowed upstairs or if I just preferred to be down there, but all of my memories of Pansy are in that walk out basement with the wood burning stove. I used to hide behind that stove and Pansy could never find me back there. I'd hide behind the hot water heater, in the dryer, behind the furniture, and under the stairs. If she couldn't find me she would start to whimper, breaking my 5-year-old little heart, so I would come out from wherever I was hiding to console her. She trained me well.

In the spring, just before I turned six, I noticed Pansy was slowing down and getting kind of fat. She wouldn't chase me like she used to and she would often lie down and pant. I was worried, so, with as much courage as I could muster, I told my mom that Pansy was acting funny and braced myself for bad news. My grandma had just been quite ill and had been acting the same way Pansy was acting, so I assumed the news was going to be bad.

My mom sat me down and told me that Pansy was pregnant and was going to have puppies. She continued to explain, but I have no idea what she said because she lost me at the word *puppies*. From then on the first question I asked each morning was, "Is Pansy going to have her puppies today?" I asked my mom every day and the answer was always the same, "Not today, Holly." Some days that answer had a little bit more attitude than other days.

I wasn't supposed to sleep in the basement with Pansy and I don't recall her being allowed upstairs. Nevertheless, my mom was not surprised to find me asleep on the couch in the basement with Pansy by my side. One morning she woke me up and said Pansy had given birth to one puppy and she thought the rest were on the way. I was excited but knew I had to be calm and sober in the face of a serious situation. I grabbed some towels and made Pansy a nest to lie in so she would be comfortable. But, she was having none of that. Pansy was pacing, panting and whining. I realized with a shock that having puppies was hard work.

I started to pace with her. I thought that I could ease her pain and anxiety and she would have an easier time. Not only was I empathizing, but I internalized her anxiety and made it my own.

Unsure if I was helping, I continued my mirroring of Pansy's pacing when I heard my mom gasp. I ran to her side. Behind the wood stove was a puppy, still in its pre-natal sack. I didn't understand. That wasn't a puppy. That looked like something my brother dragged out of the creek. It was gross and cold and slimy. How could that be a puppy? Puppies are warm and cuddly and smell good.

I was confused until my mom explained to me we had to clean off the sack and make the puppy breathe. I knew this was critical because she used her *Mom* voice with me. I grabbed one of the towels and my mom cleaned the puppy. She wrapped it up and then started rubbing it really hard. I thought she'd hurt the puppy, but the puppy suddenly whimpered and drew his first breath. My mom put Pansy in a box with the newborn puppy and we started to look for others. We found them in every hiding spot of mine, except inside the dryer. Pansy had given birth to seven puppies. Five of them survived with our intervention. We didn't find the other two in time.

This was my first experience with animal trauma. I didn't understand what would make a momma dog not take care of her puppies properly. My mom explained that sometimes first-time momma dogs don't know what to do and we had to show her. She told me that by having the puppies in my favorite hiding spots, Pansy was asking for our help. That's when I figured out dogs are very smart and could tell us what they need if we only listened.

While I was thrilled that we had five new puppies in our midst, my mind kept going back to the two we hadn't found in time. I can still recall, in detail, where those two puppies were located and what they looked like. I still feel the hole in my stomach when I think about what my 5-year-old self had to process at that moment. When I tried to talk about it with my parents, I was told that it happens sometimes and just enjoy the puppies that survived. I tried to push the graphic images out of my head and I didn't tell my parents about the nightmares I was having. I did get in trouble when I wouldn't eat. I couldn't eat. I was obsessed with the thoughts of those two puppies.

In hindsight, I understand that I was experiencing a trauma and the aftershocks of trauma. At five, I wasn't equipped to handle it. The trauma presented as bad dreams and monsters under my bed. I needed a night light for the first time in my life. I was easily annoyed. My brother constantly picked on me, so I hit him in the head with a toy gun, inflicting a gash on his head that required stitches. I was anxious and found myself going in the basement to count the puppies as soon as I got home from school every day.

If we had cell phones back then, I am sure I would have been texting my mom all morning to get reassurance that Pansy and the puppies were healthy. Instead, I developed upset tummies; so much so that my mom had to take me to the doctor. He gave my mom some little orange pills that tasted like sugar. Whenever my tummy got upset, my mom gave me one of those little pills. I have no idea what they were, and I don't even remember if they helped, but it was the only way for me to reach out to an adult and tell them I was having trouble. No one associated the death of those two puppies to my behavior and anxiety.

For the next six weeks, my mom and I took care of Pansy and her puppies, showing them how to nurse, how to huddle up for warmth and reassuring Pansy she was being a good mom. Of course, I named them all. Pansy, the five puppies and I would spend hours playing in the basement, but I avoided the areas where the two puppies had died. Those areas were cold, dark, and scary.

As the puppies grew and got more playful, I was in heaven. We went for walks in the gully, we had tea parties and I even put the puppies in my doll's clothes so they would stay warm. I cleaned up the newspapers after they had soiled them. I learned how and why Pansy licked the puppies. How she showed them how to eat hard food. How each noise that she made from a murmur to a growl meant something to those puppies. They understood and reacted to her. I got to witness their ears open up and how they would listen to all of the new sounds around them. I watched them open their little cloudy blue eyes and take a look at the world. I watched them learn to crawl, then walk, and finally romp. I explained everything to them about the world and how I would keep them safe and happy all of their lives.

Unbeknownst to me, the puppies were destined for other homes and other families who would love them and raise them. I don't recall the day I found out they were leaving, but I do remember the day that they left. Five different families came to our house. I sat on the same white concrete porch, which seemed to have turned gray, and watched one family after another go into our basement and come out with one of Pansy's puppies. I could see the happiness and excitement in their faces. Even the puppy's faces showed more curiosity than fear or heartbreak. I wasn't sure how I felt about it. Weren't they going to miss Pansy and me?

I wasn't allowed in the basement until the last puppy had gone to their new home. Pansy and I sat together for a long time, her head in my lap. I just petted her smooth head and tangled my fingers in her curly ears. I wasn't sure if I needed to say I'm sorry or not, so I just sat with her. I felt that I had betrayed her by letting her puppies go to other families. I let her sleep with her head in my lap. I missed dinner because I refused to wake her up. When she whimpered in her sleep I assumed she was crying for her puppies, which broke my little heart and I cried. I let the tears fall down my face and into Pansy's chocolate-colored curls. I was with her a long time and eventually fell asleep.

When I woke up, there was a tennis ball on my lap and a very happy Pansy ready to play. The lesson I learned from Pansy would carry into my future and help me through a difficult time in my life. She was telling me it was okay. The puppies were safe and happy and she was fine. We could enjoy the moment and play a good game of fetch. Pansy was living in the present and didn't seem haunted by the past, or by the loss of her puppies like I was. Dogs are amazing creatures. I loved Pansy and knew her attitude was a telling example that I wanted to follow.

If Not for Pets

When I was eight, we moved to a house on the shore of Lake Huron. I was thrilled to live on the beach but really struggled to make friends. Being the new kid on the block, I got picked on often. Two of the older girls decided to initiate me into the neighborhood by beating me up. One held my arms behind my back, while the other pummeled me with punches. Then they swapped places. I was too small to do anything about it and being restrained, I couldn't really fight back. After I had endured the beating, I went home and told my mom. I could tell she was hesitant to do anything about it, but she confronted the girls' mothers.

The girls denied it, which caused a bad situation for my mom and the mom of one of the girls. My mom endured her own battle with bullying by that woman the entire time we lived on the lake. I blamed myself for a long time, feeling guilt that I had to drag my mom into a battle that I believed was mine, not hers. I was beginning to cultivate an overdeveloped sense of responsibility.

Until that time, I had never been bullied by anyone other than my brother. I was assured that these girls wouldn't beat me up again, but they did. It continued until I moved away when I was 17. Being a victim of bullying needs to be addressed and supported, but back then, it was either be a victim or be the bully. I was always the victim. It was so intense, that I refused to visit the restroom in junior high or high school unless I could get out of class to do so. I suffered from anxiety and panic attacks as early as 6th grade.

I was insecure and assumed people wanted to hurt me, so learning to let people into my world was excruciating. A classmate's birthday party, sleepovers, school dances and after school sports were riddled with anxiety. My anxiety manifested itself in sleeplessness, bouts of vomiting causing weight loss, inability to be still, preoccupation with my surroundings and general fear that I was going to be hurt by someone unseen. I suffered these symptoms in silence.

My family was no help. My mom was going through her own challenges and my Dad was working. My brother only contributed to my anxiety by bullying me at home. However, when I was with a dog, all of my symptoms would dissipate. I felt safe. It felt like putting cool water on a sunburn; a complete sense of relief and calm. I sought the company of dogs. Being in the company of a dog, running my hands through its fur, looking into its eyes gave me a sense of peace, even if just for a minute or two. I believed the dogs understood that I felt better in their company, or that I needed their presence because dogs were drawn to me and seemed to seek me out. I didn't know it at the time, but this was a gift.

To this day, stray dogs just show up, even when I'm on vacation. Many times I've found a dog, with no tags, no collar, no chip and I've taken them home and cared for them until I've found their owner. Countless times a dog has dragged its owner to meet me. I always oblige by sitting in the grass with the dog, rubbing his or her ears or belly, while chatting with the owner. Many times I have heard an owner say "Wow! My dog really likes you!" or "My dog never acts like that." I have a friend who calls me the "Real Dog Whisperer" because he seems to think I can read a dog's mind. I have told him repeatedly that I can instinctively read a dog's body language, but he chooses to believe the magic, so I let him.

I learned to tread lightly when around the neighborhood kids and found solace walking on the beach by myself. I had two trusted friends, but they weren't fond of each other, so I had to divide my time between the two of them. I made friends with many of the older residents in our neighborhood and, of course, all of the dogs.

Across the street lived two big hound dogs that were trained to hunt. They lived in an outdoor kennel and I would go visit them often. Billy and Sam were always happy to see me and soon their Dad allowed me to go into their kennel to play. He even supplied me with treats to give the boys when I would go visit. Billy and Sam's Dad told his friends in our neighborhood about me and my love of his dogs. He looked upon his dogs as tools. I looked upon them as friends. He taught me how to train them. I taught him how to love them. In their elder years, they became house dogs.

We had lived on the lake for about two years when an older lady who lived down the street needed a baby sitter for her Jack Russell Terrier, Sparky. She was friends with Billy and Sam's dad so she asked my parents if I could watch her dog. I was delighted when my parents said I could. I went over to her house on a Friday afternoon and she walked me through everything I needed to know to take care of Sparky. I was scheduled to spend four hours with him the next day starting at 10 am. What a gig!

I was so excited I couldn't sleep that Friday night and when 9:45 am rolled around, I left the house and ran to Sparky's house. His mom was very kind and left a Coke and some macaroni and cheese for me for lunch in the fridge. She'd be home by 2:00 pm and I only had to walk him once. We went out for a walk just before noon and ran right smack into the neighborhood bullies. I froze. My flight or fight response was immediately activated. My biggest worry was they would hurt Sparky. Surprisingly, I realized I would fight to protect this little dog in my charge. Sparky gave them a bit of growl and they moved right along. I inwardly smiled for this victory over the bullies with the help of this little dog.

This incident cemented my belief that I was safe if I were with a dog. After our walk, we enjoyed our lunch together and then watched cartoons on TV. It was a gray, late autumn day and the lake was starting to get rough as the north wind started to blow, so spending time in the house seemed like a great idea and I knew we were safe.

When his mom came home, I told her about our day and she offered to drive me home. I didn't know at the time that she knew about the bullies and was trying to keep me safe. When we got to my driveway, she handed me $20 and asked if I'd be willing to watch Sparky again. I said, "Of course!" So began my career as a professional pet sitter. I'd get to watch Sparky one Saturday a month for four hours while his mom ran her errands in town. The town was over 30 minutes away, so she only liked to drive that far once a month.

I truly enjoyed my time with Sparky. I felt safe with him, unlike when I was on my own; safer than I felt in my own home. I had the privilege of pet sitting for Sparky every Saturday for about a year. While that may not seem like a long time, I calculated it in dog years. So, I had known Sparky for seven years. Taking care of Sparky taught me that it was okay to be alone as long as I had a dog with me. It taught me how to properly care for someone else's pet, while instilling in me an unbeatable work ethic. It taught me to be respectful of other people's homes and privacy and set me up for a prosperous pet sitting career later in life.

Sparky's mom developed a serious illness and her kids had to help her move out of her home and into assisted living. Unfortunately, she couldn't take Sparky with her. This was distressing and I empathized with her pain of losing her dog. I tried to help by asking my parents if he could come and live with us. They said no, but I kept trying to find him a home. I was not successful and felt like I had failed Sparky and his mom. My overdeveloped sense of responsibility was growing and would fuel my actions for the next several decades.

I missed Sparky and our time together, but I had learned being with dogs was where I wanted to be.

First Love

When we moved to the lake, my parents promised me that I could get a dog of my own. It took a few years for them to fulfill this promise, but they did. On a warm spring day, my Dad brought home a young Alaskan Malamute whom I immediately named Toots. The promise of a new furry best friend filled my brain and, within seconds, I envisioned her sleeping in my bed at night, listening intently while I read her books and told her stories. She'd go walking the beach with me. I thought she'd be the dog who would wait at the end of the driveway for me every day when the school bus dropped me off. She'd be my Lassie and I'd be her Timmy. These thoughts swirled through my head within seconds of my Dad putting this puffball of a dog into my arms. I had my head buried in her neck, murmuring words of immediate love and gratitude towards this dog. She responded to me and nestled up against me and heaved a big sigh. She was my first heart dog.

While Toots and I were falling in puppy love, my Dad was getting things out of the back of his work truck. He was a carpenter, so the rattling of tools was normal and no cause for alarm, until I realized that he was pulling a chain out of his truck. Then, he heaved a massive dog house out of his truck along with a metal bowl and some carpeting. I didn't understand. When I asked him about it, he said it was Toot's doghouse and she would be living outside, chained, next to the garage. I was immediately heartbroken. Even though I tried to argue the point vigorously, my Dad had his mind made up and Toots was destined to be an outdoor dog.

I may have been a Daddy's girl, but this was a battle I wasn't going to win and I knew it. I was disappointed and felt a burden of responsibility. I believed that I had to make it up to her. I projected my expected ideals unto her and figured she felt the same way. When my Dad put the chain around her neck and snapped the other end to her doghouse, it felt like a jail cell door slamming closed. I could feel my hands balling up into little fists and the compulsion to fight for a better life for this dog, but I was 10 and I had no real power or authority.

I wrestled with the feeling of inadequacy for several weeks while I spent time with Toots outside. I taught her to "sit" and "shake" and "speak", but she was on a chain and I felt more like her keeper than her friend. Finally, I realized that I was fighting a losing battle with my Dad to let her be a house dog. I made up my mind to make the best of it for Toots' sake, and mine.

It wasn't the ideal situation for the dog, or for me, but she was counting on me to take care of her and I took that seriously. Every morning I would feed her and give her fresh water before I left for school. On the few occasions I forgot because I was running late for school, I felt such shame and grief that I couldn't get home fast enough. Twice, I made my mom come and get me from school, feigning illness, because I couldn't handle the guilt. It was a huge weight for a preteen. It never occurred to me to just ask my mom to feed and water Toots. I shouldered the burden, anthropomorphized Toots' feelings, and continued to build my overdeveloped sense of responsibility for her.

Toots grew quickly and I loved having a big dog. Her doghouse was large enough to house both of us. I stashed a flashlight inside, so I could climb in and read my current Nancy Drew or Tiger Beat to her. With her large head in my lap, I would tell her stories and secrets and pet her. I guess my parents assumed I was out playing with the neighborhood kids, but I spent a lot of my time in the dog house with Toots. She lacked for nothing in my power to provide. I used my allowance money to buy her treats. When I was lucky, I convinced the butcher who lived up the street to bring home a bone for her. I tried to groom her, but she wasn't fond of the brush, and I completely understood her disdain. I hated it when my mom brushed my hair, too.

As Toots grew, it didn't dawn on me to check the chain around her neck. I realized one day that her neck had grown around her chain. I was horrified. Her skin had just absorbed the chain and it was becoming part of her neck. I was mortified and riddled with guilt. How could I have missed such a thing? It had to hurt her, but Toots gave no indication that she was even bothered. However, I knew this required immediate intervention, so I burst into the house and, in a tone thick with recrimination, informed my parents what had happened.

My Dad was the first to his feet, and his reaction reinforced my belief that this was urgent. We ran outside while my mom called the vet. I remember vividly, my Dad kneeling down next to this huge dog, and gently brushing her fur away from her neck to see how bad things really were. When he hung his head, I knew it was bad. I found myself reassuring my Dad while we raced off to the veterinarian. I had one hand on his shoulder and the other hand on Toots' head, telling them both that we were all going to be okay and apologizing that I hadn't caught it sooner. The vet met us at the door and took Toots to the back of the clinic immediately. The feeling of uselessness was immediate and shocking and I wasn't sure how to handle it; so I paced and paced. Feeling anxious and unsafe, I braced myself so I wouldn't cry and remained strong for the sake of my dog.

What seemed like hours later, the vet returned my dog to us, explaining the chain had only grown under a thin layer of skin and it was easily removed without complications or stitches. She gave my Dad a stern talking to about the use of a collar versus the chain and shot me a wink as she did so. I took note of that wink, as the glimmer of realization took hold in my brain that maybe there were other people in the world who felt about dogs the same way I did. We took Toots home with a brand new red collar and I felt a bit vindicated. She was still chained to the doghouse, but occasionally I would catch my Dad out there, petting her and talking to her.

Taking Toots for a walk was my favorite thing to do. I didn't have a leash for her, so I would unclip her chain from her doghouse, wind it up around my hand and take off for an adventure. Toots loved the beach and seemed to have a gift for finding the smelliest, nastiest things to roll in. She also loved to pull. I knew Malamutes were sled dogs and I had no idea how to make her stop pulling me except to dig in and hold on. She outweighed me by about 20 pounds and the sheer torque of her strength would usually land me on my butt. As soon as I hit the ground, she would turn around and tackle me.

It was sheer joy; until my parents found out what I was doing. They forbade me walking her. My Dad knew how stubborn I was going to be on this particular subject because he knew how much I loved spending time with Toots, so he made sure he chose the most gruesome, graphic example of what could happen if I foolishly decided to walk my dog. He tried to tell me it was dangerous and I could get hurt. She could get away from me and get hit by a car (he provided me with horrific details) or run away and *never come back*. Undeterred, I walked my dog when my parents weren't home. Toots deserved to explore and enjoy adventures and I was confident in my ability to handle her. We continued to enjoy the beach and the gully and the field across the street, and my upper body strength began to develop and grow.

Soon, I wasn't landing on my butt as much when she began to pull and I was learning how to tell her not to pull. She was a very good teacher and was truly patient with me. The chain was the biggest issue and I was struggling to find a way to handle the chain without pain in my hands. But I persisted. My hands became rough and calloused, my arms became solid with muscle and my shoulders gained strength. Toots and I were a good team.

My only wish was for a leash. The clip of the chain would dig into my hands when Toots would pull and one hot summer day on our way to the water, the clip of the chain caught the inside of my finger right at the middle knuckle and dug down to the bone. It hurt like heck and there was blood everywhere.   I continued to the water so Toots could get a drink and enjoy the coolness of the lake on a hot summer day. I put my hand in the water to take the heat out of the injury and assess the damage. It looked kind of bad, but if I put a band aid on it with some Neosporin, the flap of skin would reattach and my finger would heal up just fine.

Two days later I woke up to a finger the size of a sausage. I couldn't move it and it was red, hot and angry. I took the band aid off, which hurt so much I nearly passed out. My knuckle was so swollen that my finger wouldn't bend, no matter how hard I tried. It wasn't bleeding but there were red streaks running down my finger and into my hand. My stomach was upset and my muscles ached all over. I knew it was time to tell my parents what had happened. I knew I was going to get a licking for disobeying them, but I'd have to face my punishment in order to get help.

My fear of going to them wasn't for my own punishment, in as much as it was for Toots. I went to her first, showed her my finger and explained to her that I had to tell my parents what had happened. She sniffed my finger, looked me right in the eye, and slowly hung her head. I knew what she said and what she wanted me to do.

I was frightened, but boldly went to my mom and showed her my finger. The look of horror on her face when she saw my finger only solidified the fact that I had done the right thing by coming to her. I knew my knuckle was in trouble. I wasn't sure about my personal standing at that moment, but it didn't seem to matter that I had disobeyed my parents because I was in the Emergency Room within 30 minutes. I got a shot in the hip, which hurt as much as my finger, an IV full of fluid and antibiotics. A kind and caring nurse came in and managed to clean my knuckle without me passing out. I was sent home the next day with 21 days of antibiotics, instructions to keep the dressing dry and the wound clean. I knew the importance of following these directions because the doctor said if I didn't I could lose my finger.

This distressed me because I had just learned how to use that finger to flip off my brother when he started to harass me. He didn't know about my hiding spot in Toot's doghouse, so my courage had started to grow in defending myself against him.

I spent the next 21 days following Doctor's orders and didn't lose my finger. I anticipated a harsh punishment from my parents and was imagining the worse when I got called downstairs to talk about it. I always knew I was in big trouble when my Dad would start a sentence with "And the next time I tell you to do something...." Or "I'm so disappointed in you", which actually hurt worse than any physical punishment he gave. Feeling impending doom, tears already rolling down my cheeks, I faced my parents. I lifted my chin and tried to be brave and accept responsibility for my actions. I was utterly speechless when, instead of giving me a licking, they gave me a red leash.

The following summer, my mom decided to get two pet rabbits. I don't remember her reason for getting the rabbits, but we had just read <u>Watership Down</u>, so we named the rabbits Fiver and BigWig. They were housed in a small hutch in the garage but were free range during the day. A big black rabbit and a smaller white rabbit would happily roam our yard, munching on dandelion greens and leaving small pellets in their wake. Toots loved to snack on those pellets, much to my disgust.

I was fond of the rabbits and would spend time with them, but they weren't affectionate, as rabbits go, and I didn't feel a tight bond with them. I loved having them around, though, and Fiver was my favorite. I was tasked with their housing arrangements, meaning I had to let them out in the morning and herd them at night. Have you ever tried to herd a rabbit? I honestly think this chore was more for the amusement of my parents than the safety of the rabbits. Their hutch had a tricky latch, and occasionally it wouldn't close completely and they would get out and explore the garage at night. They found great spots to hide in the debris of the garage and then I would leave the garage door ajar in the morning, so they could get out for their daily rabbit shenanigans.

While the rabbits lived with us, I continued to walk Toots. We worked on her not pulling me and basic commands. I had no idea I was actually training her, I just thought I was teaching her some manners so she wouldn't hurt me. As a full grown Malamute, she weighed in at over 100 pounds, while I barely weighed 70, so manners were essential.

One early autumn afternoon, Toots and I were out gallivanting, as usual, when she stopped at the garage to sniff. She was very intent on whatever it was on the other side of the door, and really seemed to be enjoying herself, so I indulged her. It was early afternoon and the breeze was still warm from the last vestiges of summer. The leaves were just starting to turn and the air was crisper, so I assumed Toots was sniffing the change of seasons. The lawn mower had been used the day before and my brother hadn't rinsed it off like he had been told, so when Toots asked to go into the garage, I didn't think twice. I opened the door for her and she took off like a shot. The leash was ripped right out of my hand and she disappeared around the other side of the lawn mower. I wasn't sure what had gotten her so excited, but I quickly shut the door so she couldn't get out of the garage. There was complete darkness in the windowless garage. I could hear Toots rummaging with great intent near the lawn mower, but I couldn't see what she was doing.

Then I heard the scream. Fiver was under the lawn mower, probably munching on freshly cut grass. It was day time. She was supposed to be outside, not in the garage. I didn't know I could move so fast, but I was at Toots' side in an instant. I wasn't fast enough. She had Fiver by the head in her mouth and gave her one good shake. I instinctively grabbed Toots' snout and told her to let go in the biggest voice I could find. Startled by my harsh tone, she did let go. I scooped Fiver up into my arms as my brother came running into the garage. I told him to go take Toots back to her doghouse as I rushed into the house to my mom covered in blood, holding her rabbit.

At this point, I'm not sure what my poor mom was thinking, considering my escapades of late, but she gathered her wits and we headed to the veterinarian. It was the same veterinarian who had winked at me when Toots was treated for her ingrown chain. The kind-hearted vet took Fiver, whom I had wrapped in a towel, out of my hands, put her hand on my shoulder and told me she would do the best she could to save Fiver's life.

When she had gone, my mom finally asked me what happened. It wasn't until that moment I realized it was completely my fault. I had opened the door. I had let Toots in the garage. I had closed the door and Fiver had no escape. I felt tremendous guilt, and try as she might, my mom could not alleviate it. As we sat and waited for the vet, my mind kept going over the details of what had happened. I tried to think of a way I could have done it differently. I started pacing and got lost in my thoughts. The sights, the sounds, the smells were indelibly burned into my brain and I was having a hard time staying present with my mom. I couldn't form words to describe what was happening to me. Instead, I continued to pace while my mom tried to get me to talk. I felt that if I even opened my mouth to speak, I would vomit. While I now know these are the early stages of shock, this event ultimately led to nightmares, intrusive graphic images and a preoccupation with the event. A pre-teen's version of PTSD and it wouldn't be the last time I suffered from it.

Soon the vet came out to see us and with a distressed look on her face, explained to us the damage Toots had inflicted. Toots had grabbed Fiver by the head, breaking her skull and damaging her brain. She believed the injury was survivable, but Fiver would be in pain the rest of her life and had irreversible brain damage. She looked at me and said, "Young lady, you have two choices. I can do the best I can for your bunny, but she will never be the same and will

34

have pain the rest of her life. Or, I can put her to sleep right now and relieve her suffering. What would you like me to do?" I looked at my mom, who urged me to make the decision.

This was my first glimpse of the killing/caring paradox in animal care. We, as pet owners, pet caretakers and pet professionals, are tasked with the unique and unenviable decision of ending a life that we have intimately cared for. As an adult, this decision is difficult at best, but as a child, it seemed nearly impossible. However, my response to the veterinarian was almost immediate and I said to her, "Please, don't let her suffer. I'm sorry. It's my fault."

The vet nodded her head and turned to walk away and I said to her, "Could I please have her tail?" Morbid, maybe, but even today I can't tell you what motivated me to ask for her tail. I needed to have it. I kept it for many years until I lost it in a fire that destroyed our house when I was 18. I also spent several years volunteering my time on Saturdays and Wednesday afternoons with that same veterinarian to learn how to properly care for animals. I had made too many mistakes already and I wanted, no needed, to learn how to care for my animals properly.

Toots lived to the ripe old dog age of 13. When I moved out on my own with Tony (my husband) Toots came with me. Together, we were able to finally give her the house dog life I had so desperately wanted to give her when I was a kid. BigWig, the rabbit, passed away shortly after we lost Fiver. I believe he died of a broken heart over losing his sister. I continued to blame myself, not Toots, for Fiver's death.

I relived the event over and over in my head for a very long time. To this day, fresh-cut grass reminds me of that day. The scent of the early autumn or the feel of the warm breeze right after summer as the leaves change will alter my mood without warning. While these experiences become diluted with time, each one of them contributed to my becoming a professional pet sitter and my battle with compassion fatigue.

Traumatic events, ones that burn themselves into the brain, are fodder for significant mental distress later in life. They are stored in the memory, to be relived when conditions are right. It's called Primary Trauma and can lead to PTSD (Post Traumatic Stress Disorder). Compassion fatigue is cumulative and this was just the beginning for me. I'm resilient and appeared to bounce back from these tragic events. However, my behavior during my early teens was self-destructive and reckless. I struggled with my own form of PTSD well into my teenage years. I continued to view the world as a dangerous place and assumed there was always a bad guy in the bushes.

Rescuing Animals – Saving Me

When I was 13, I got a job as a weekend dishwasher at a small local restaurant. It gave me something to focus on and a place to expend my anxious energy. I was a great dishwasher. I didn't meet a dried-fried-egg plate I couldn't scrub clean. Work became my coping mechanism and I started to feel like I had some control. Work became my counsel, my outlet, and my proving ground. My work ethic was rewarded and applauded, so it grew and flourished.

I remember we had an outdoor cat named Mabel. I don't recall the exact details of her coming into our family, but I do remember she was a sweet, gray striped tabby with a white belly and white socks. I hated that she was banished from the house, but my Dad said he was allergic to cats. Winters in Michigan are brutal, especially on Lake Huron, and I could not handle the thought of Mabel suffering outside in the cold.

The first few times I snuck her into my room, I actually went outside and brought her inside in my jacket. I had a litter box set up in my closet and food and water under my bed. My parents didn't come into my room often and I had a lock on my door to keep my brother out, so no one was the wiser. I'd go get her after dinner and hide her in my room until morning. Then I would shoo her out the window so she could spend the day outside doing whatever it was she did during the day. It didn't take long before she started showing up at my window at night to come in. It was the perfect set up and it went on for several years. Mabel would only come to my window when it was cold or storming, otherwise, she stayed outside. I loved it when she came in. She'd sleep with me. The weight of her body on my feet was reassuring and comforting.

While the cat was playing stowaway in my room during these years, a wonderful part Golden Retriever with white boots showed up on our back porch one day. She was a house dog and there was no getting around that fact. She was also heavy with puppies. Between my Mom and me, my Dad didn't stand a chance. He finally relented and let her in one of the rooms by the back door. When he agreed to let the dog come in the house, I was elated.

I named this wonderful dog Boots. Between Mabel and Boots being in the house, I didn't spend much time away from home. Boots had come to us in her time of need and I wasn't going to be the one to send her away, so my mom and I made a nice room for her and took her and Toots for walks. As she got heavier with puppies, she slowed down and soon I had to leave her behind when Toots and I went out for walks.

One day, I came home from school and there were puppies—12 of them. Boots had delivered all 12 puppies just like a Momma dog should and by the time I got home, they were clean, squirmy and lively. It dawned on me just how worried I had been about Boots giving birth, given that my only other experience was with Pansy and her puppies. I was relieved that things had gone well. Boots was happy and healthy and we had 12 puppies to care for. I brought Toots in to see the puppies but she turned her nose up at them. I assumed she felt about puppies the way I felt about babies and I didn't hold it against her. The puppies ate and slept and grew and grew.

This time, I was prepared for them to be given to other families, but I assumed I'd get to keep Boots. I was wrong. My Dad made arrangements for Boots to go to a farm after her puppies had been given to other homes. My mom managed to talk him into keeping two of her puppies. It still amazes me that she was able to do it. The farmer came and got Boots and put her in the trunk of his car and took her away. The fact that he put her in the trunk caused me great distress. I felt I had let down another dog. Although I was distraught, I consoled myself with the two puppies.

My mom named them Weasel and Wooly Bear. They were completely different. Weasel was a reddish-golden puppy, while Wooly Bear was black and white. Weasel was huge and Wooly Bear was tiny. Weasel was outgoing and happy while Wooly Bear was reserved and unsure of herself. The theory was the Boots had two baby daddies resulting in two litters being born at the same time. The vet assured me this was possible but uncommon. Looking at the puppies, I knew it was true. They were an unlikely and inseparable pair.

As Weasel and Wooly Bear grew, my mom was their primary caregiver. I still walked Toots and took care of her. I had noticed that Mabel was getting slow and eating less. I couldn't tell my parents or they would have figured out she was hiding in my room, so I spoke to the veterinarian who had helped me earlier. She gave me the information I needed to tend to Mabel, who, by now, spent most of her time on my bed.

I didn't have much input when it came to the puppies. They were definitely Mom's dogs and she developed an unyielding attachment to them that I didn't understand at the time. I loved those two pups, but they were in tune with my mom and vice versa. Mabel's health steadily declined and she rarely went outside anymore. My Dad spent less and less time at home and my mom and the puppies were in their own world. My brother had left for the Army and I thought the puppies were helping Mom through her grief. Then, my mom started spending less time at home as well. I was left to tend to all of the animals on my own in addition to working part time, going to high school and spending time with my boyfriend. My life was plenty busy.

The End of Family As I Knew It

On a cold weekend in March, my Dad said he was going skiing with some friends. My mom didn't accompany him. I had to work all weekend and had plans with my boyfriend. Mabel wasn't doing well, but she continued to eat and use her box, so I wasn't overly concerned about her. My mom was devoted to her two new dogs and didn't seem to care that Mabel was in the house when she discovered my secret that weekend. Monday morning rolled around and my Dad wasn't back yet. I ate my breakfast, fed and watered Toots, fed and watered Mabel, and left for school. When I got home two distressing matters awaited me.

First, Mabel had passed away on my bed in her sleep. I discovered her as I dropped my books on my bed. I had been summoned downstairs by my parents and was torn as to what to do. I wrapped her body in a towel and took it downstairs with me. As I stood there, holding my lifeless cat, already in tears, my Dad informed me he was leaving my mom and me. He had filed for divorce and was moving out that day.

Things with my parents finally made sense. I felt relief and validation for knowing that there really was something wrong. I remember falling to my knees in despair, but it wasn't because my Dad was leaving. It was because Mabel had died. I felt I had let down another animal. I don't remember much else about that day except I made up my mind not to let down any more animals if I had the power to do better.

Our life dramatically changed after my Dad left. My mom spent less and less time at home and developed a bar hopping habit. My Dad was busy rebuilding his life. With my brother gone, I spent a lot of time alone at home with the dogs. As Weasel and Wooly Bear got older, they became good listeners and great house dogs. On cold winter nights, I would bring Toots in the house to sleep. With three big dogs in the house, I felt physically safe in my home even though I was alone.

As drinking often does, it took over my mom's life. When it started to intrude on my life, I sought help — all I could find; professional help, support groups and personal mentors. While I wasn't crazy about the idea of verbally vomiting on people, I knew that I had to share my past traumas and the current drama in my home in order to move forward. I didn't want to get stuck in the mire of addiction, but it was hard to move ahead because my mom was suffering. Letting go comes at a price. The price is usually guilt and shame and I was carrying a suitcase full of both.

As I worked through this process, Pansy came to mind. I remembered how she had to let go of her puppies. I remembered how she gave herself time to grieve and then moved forward. I took it a bit further and assumed that she let herself enjoy her life after her puppies left. So, that's what I decided to do, at the age of 18.

With the help of many people, I was able to finally talk about the traumas I had endured and had a safe place to share the drama that was my current life. My mom descended further into addiction. Meanwhile, my Dad rented out our home for the summer for a bit of extra income. Strangers would be enjoying our home on the lake and we would live in a small house Dad rented for us. It was both distressing and a relief to me at the same time.

My mom and I had about half of our things moved into the new home when she decided to stop for the night. The dogs were still at the house on the lake, so I got in my car and went and got them. I didn't want to spend the night alone. My mom went out with her friends while I stayed at the new house with the dogs and some MTV.

MTV was a novelty at the new house. We didn't have access to cable up on the lake, so when I found out I could have my MTV, I was glued to the couch to watch the videos. I fell asleep on the couch with the dogs by my side. I don't know when my mom decided to come home that night, but when I woke up my Dad was at our house. I heard the now familiar sound of his stern voice as he talked to my mom like she was a child, reprimanding her for being out so late, or so I thought.

I let the dogs out the back door, rubbed the sleep out of my eyes and went into the new kitchen to say good morning to my parents. My mom was sitting at the table with her head down and my Dad was standing over her, with his hand on her back. I couldn't come to terms with the fact that he was touching her in such an intimate way. I hadn't seen them touch since he decided to leave us. I knew he already had a girlfriend. As my tired mind tried to reconcile what I was seeing, my Dad told me to sit down. Based on the sound of his voice, I thought I was in trouble, again. I did as I was told with no questions. He shook his head as if he was at a loss for words.

I immediately started to panic. I felt my stomach get hot and the heat spread through my arms and legs. I felt dizzy. He seemed to sense he was losing me so he touched my arm and reeled me back in. He then proceeded to tell me that our house on the lake had caught fire the night before. The fire had destroyed everything we had left in the house. We only had what we had already moved to the new house. He told me that the fire was so fast and so hot, that the firefighters had told him if any living thing had been in the house at the time, they would not have made it out.

Then, he stopped and looked at me to make sure I understood what he was telling me. We were lucky to be alive and particularly lucky the dogs were with us that night in the new house. Had I not made the last trip to get them, they would have been in the house when it burned down.

I'd like to say that experience changed my mom's behavior, but it didn't. Her story is hers to tell and not mine. She made some interesting friends and introduced me to some interesting people. Had she not met one friend, in particular, I would never have met my husband, Tony.

Creating My Own Family

Mom's best friend was a lady named Cathy. She was bad news and I knew it. So did the dogs. None of us liked her, but we had to contend with her. One day, Cathy showed up with her three kids and nowhere to go, so Mom said they could stay with us for a few days. I was not happy that I had to share my tiny bedroom with two girls I barely knew. Cathy slept on the floor in Mom's room. Glen, her son, slept on the couch. I was upset because there wasn't any room for Weasel and Wooly Bear and I had trouble sleeping without them.

During the day everyone scattered, so I had the luxury of a few hours to myself with the dogs. I vividly remember sitting on the living room floor, painting my nails with the dogs at my feet when Glen walked in the living room followed by one of his friends. The dogs picked up their heads, so I turned my head and met the gaze of this tall, willowy young man with dark hair and a great pair of Levi's. It was an immediate spark, for me at least. I can't remember much else about what happened that day, except to say that Tony drove me to work. He had an old, green 69 Buick LeSabre with a bench seat in the front and I had to sit in the middle because he refused to move his cassette tapes from the passenger seat. I guess he felt that spark too.

Three days later, I broke off my engagement to my high school boyfriend and began a lifelong love affair with Tony. The best part about him (besides the great pair of Levi's) was his love for my dogs—especially Toots, whom he affectionately called Tootsie Bear.

Tony and I have been inseparable ever since. We've gone through some troubling times, but we've stuck together. If it weren't for him and his constant support and love, I wouldn't have made it through most of my pet sitting career. We've learned how to let go of things we thought we needed, learned how to grow up and be responsible adults, brought a child into the world and, hopefully, raised him to be a contributing, responsible adult in his own right. And through it all, we loved each other.

Toots came with me when I married Tony, but after her passing we lived without a dog. While I loved being married, I wanted a dog in the worst way. I was pet sitting a big Samoyed named Bear on weekends. Tony would pick him up from his parent's house on Fridays after work and bring him home so I could take care of him all weekend. Then, on Mondays, Tony would drop him back off at his house.

Eventually, his parents decided to let me keep him and I was thrilled. Bear was my heart dog and he knew I was pregnant before I did! He started sleeping on my side of the bed at night, instead of in his crate and followed me all over the house. So, when we found out I was pregnant, Bear looked at me as if to say, "See? I told you!"

My pregnancy was far from easy. Premature labor started when I was only three months along. I can remember bending over to get the laundry out of the dryer and I'd have contractions. Twice I was hospitalized for premature labor, finally forcing my Doctor to put me on bed rest for 16 weeks. I couldn't walk my dog, couldn't take care of my dog except to let him out when I was allowed off of the couch for 10 minutes every hour. That was just enough time for the dog and me to do our respective business and get a drink before we had to head back to the couch. Those 16 weeks were terribly boring, but I was growing a human and needed to rest.

Bear started to get restless. I thought he was bored, like I was, and needed more attention. Tony did his best to take care of me and the dog, but something wasn't right with Bear. He started to get really slow. He didn't want his hind end rubbed or his back feet touched. He wouldn't let me brush him and his appetite waned. Sensing serious trouble, I crawled under the dining room table one day, which wasn't

49

easy, to have a chat with him. I wanted to know what was wrong. I thought it was the impending birth; maybe he was feeling insecure or jealous. Not knowing exactly what was wrong, I reached out to pet him. Once again, one of my best friends bit me — right on my arm. Only this time it wasn't a warning, Bear meant it. He was in pain and didn't want me touching him. I heeded his bite.

I backed out from under the table, grabbed the phone and went back to the couch, hoping the contractions that had started would stop on their own. Tony rushed home from work and took Bear to the vet. After tests and x-rays, we discovered, to our dismay, that Bear was suffering stage 5 hip dysplasia. He was only three years old at the time.

I remember going to see my baby doctor and telling him what happened. He was upset by the news and concerned about my well-being because we decided to have Bear put to sleep. The vet told us he was in excruciating pain and there was nothing that could be done short of hip replacement surgery. With a baby on the way, one income and very little stability, we felt we had no option. My baby doctor told me to take it easy and try to stay calm. I didn't have much longer to go and he was encouraging me to be as quiet as I could. He understood my plight, having a Golden Retriever of his own, but was very frank about what would happen should I have the baby too early. I heeded his warning, kept myself calm and quiet and stayed on the couch.

Not being able to grieve a terrible loss is difficult. If a wave a grief washed over me and I started to cry, I'd have contractions. I'd have to stop crying which only made me want to cry harder. It took immense willpower and discipline to keep it together for the sake of our baby, alone, on the couch, without my dog for company.

Once I was released from bed rest, the first thing I did was buy a balloon full of helium. I taped Bear's picture to the balloon and wrote small notes of love and gratitude and tied them to the balloon. I stood in the back yard, with Tony, and cried for my dog. I was heartbroken. I turned my chin towards the sky and let the tears run down into my ears as I let the balloon go into the sky. I said goodbye to my heart dog that day, but never truly let him go. I still have his ashes in my treasure drawer.

Once released from bed rest, I started walking everywhere. We went to the mall just to walk around. We went to the beach to walk. I didn't feel a contraction for two weeks after I got off of the couch. Cyle was two weeks late. However, when he did decide it was time to enter the world, it took two hours, three big pushes and one dislocated shoulder on his part. Tony and I had a baby boy, born in 1992, weighing in at nearly 10 pounds.

The Family is Complete

Our family couldn't be complete without a dog and we picked an Alaskan Malamute puppy named Glace (rhymes with lacy) Mae out of a litter of 11. Our landlord, at the time, was a prize-winning Alaskan Malamute Breeder and was dedicated to the breed and the authenticity of the bloodline. One of her dogs was actually a European Grand Champion, but at the time I was more impressed with his sheer size. He weighed about 130 pounds and was magnificent. I believed he was what an Alaskan Malamute should look like. He had a long, wooly coat and a black mask around his eyes that made him look like a bandit. His ears were soft as velvet and he would fold them back into an aerodynamic tuck when he ran, his fur rippling in the wind. He was Glace Mae's grandpa.

When we first brought Glace Mae home, Tony and our landlord decided that they wanted Glace to be a show dog. Tony spent hours learning how to handle Glace in the show ring. He learned how to stack her, run with her and groom her until her coat glistened. They were showing in the puppy class with the goal of awards, medals and titles as she grew.

I was not interested in having a show dog, but Tony seemed to be enjoying the experience and so did Glace. By the time she was eight months old, however, the judges said she was "too big" to be a show dog by their standards. They preferred petite Malamutes. I did not, and I did not appreciate that some judge could arbitrarily say that my dog didn't fit the standards. I felt that Malamutes should be big dogs. Glace Mae was nearly 80 pounds already. Attributing human emotions to my dog wasn't new for me, so I assumed she took this slight as personally as I did. I was sure her feelings were hurt so, unbeknownst to my landlord and my husband; I had Glace Mae spayed, which effectively took her out of competitions. We wouldn't have to worry about what judges thought about my dog anymore.

I know Glace Mae loved me and Cyle, but her heart belonged to her Daddy. She was Tony's heart dog. I was happy for Tony and for Glace Mae. After losing Bear, I felt like I'd never be ready for another heart dog. I gave my heart to Cycle and focused on being a mom.

Tony took his role as Glace Mae's leader seriously. He trained her in basic commands, took her for long walks and even taught her how to sit in Cyle's bicycle trailer. He pulled the trailer behind his bike and we all went for bike rides together. Full grown, Glace Mae weighed in at over 100 pounds. Sitting next to a toddler who was wearing a big blue helmet, in a trailer behind a bike, she drew a lot of attention. She was a patient dog and tolerant of Tony's antics. He put sunglasses on her face and took her picture. He carved a pumpkin for her one Halloween and then tried to get her to wear it on her head. He bought her Christmas gifts and special collars. He would blow in her nose and chuckle when she sneezed. He loved to pick her up and hold her like a baby. In turn, she'd lick his entire face, tail wagging with enthusiasm. This was Tony's first heart dog and it brought me such joy to see how their love for each other. She went everywhere with us.

One Saturday, we went to Canada to get some delicious fish from a little hole-in-the-wall bar. We had Cyle and Glace Mae. As we pulled into the parking lot we realized maybe the dog couldn't go into the bar with us for dinner. I tried anyway. We just walked in like we knew what we were doing and like it was totally normal for a dog to be in a bar in Canada so we could eat some fish. We almost made it to a table before someone realized there was a giant, wooly dog in the bar. We were asked politely to take the dog outside, which we did after everyone got to pet her.

We got our fish to go and headed off to the park. The fish was delicious, as one would expect from a hole-in-the-wall bar. It was even wrapped in newspaper, which Glace Mae thought would make a great snack. After we ate, we got out of the car and went for a walk. There was a small river running through the park. It was fast flowing, but crystal clear and cold. We could see the bottom of the river and fish swimming around. Apparently, Glace Mae could see the fish as well because the next thing we knew she was in the river trying to catch the fish. I heard the splash and realized the dog was gone. When she made her way back to the top of the water, she was wearing a tremendous smile, as if she had just made a wonderful discovery. Tony still had her leash in his hand and I don't know how he managed not to fall in the river when Glace dove in. We sat in the warm summer sun for quite some time while she dried off enough to put her back in the car.

A memorable exception to the rule of Glace Mae going everywhere with us was one Christmas when Cyle was a toddler. My Dad loves chocolate covered cherries and ever since I was a little girl, I had bought him chocolate covered cherries and Old Spice for Christmas. One Christmas, although finances were tight, found a way to buy presents for our family including the cherries.

After all of the presents were purchased, wrapped and placed under our Christmas tree with the utmost care, we went out for Coney Dogs. Tony and I loved Coney Dogs and it was a special treat for us. It was such an enjoyable meal we were hesitant to leave, but Cyle could only sit for so long.

We arrived home to a dark house, but no dog greeting us. If not in her crate, Glace would usually meet us at the door when we came home. I flipped on the light and noticed wrapping paper strewn all over the living room. I inwardly groaned. Upon closer inspection, I found that Glace Mae had done very little damage. She had unwrapped every single present, flung the wrapping paper around, but left the gifts untouched—except for the chocolate covered cherries.

Panic set in as raced around our little house trying to find our dog and the remains of the box of cherries. All of the terrible consequences were flashing through my mind. Would she be sick? Would she be unconscious? Did we get home in time? Will there be a veterinarian open this late? How would we pay an emergency vet bill? These questions and a million others formed in a matter of seconds as I searched for my dog.

I found her, in Cyle's room, on the floor, with the box of chocolate covered cherries between her front feet. The box was opened, but not shredded. There were two chocolate covered cherries missing and based on the chocolate and sticky goo she had on her face, she was wearing most of it. I watched her as she delicately put her snout into the box and with only her front teeth, gently grabbed a chocolate covered cherry out of the box. She put it on the ground, pushed it around with her nose, and then rolled around on it after she had licked it. She didn't know I was watching her until I started laughing out loud. We haven't put presents under the Christmas tree since that incident. For the record, I did call the veterinarian and Glace Mae was fine.

Glace Mae and Cyle were the best of friends. The three of us spent countless hours on the floor, playing with blocks, Legos and toys while watching Aladdin, over and over again. To this day, Cyle can still recite the entire movie. Glace seemed to know the difference between her toys and Cyle's and she never chewed on any of his things. There were times when they would climb in her crate together. She'd lay herself down so he had enough room and they would enjoy each other's company. Sometimes, he'd take a book with him and he would read to her. I was always close by and enjoyed just watching them together. It took me back to my childhood when I would read my books to Toots.

Glace Mae was also a chipmunk hunter. We loved to take her camping up north and watch her shove her nose down a chipmunk hole. She'd huff in the dirt, throw her head back and huff the dirt out of her nose. She'd sneeze then do it again until she had found just the right scent. Then, she'd start to dig. Her digging was joyous and when she was digging, it seemed she was fulfilling a primal need. When we would pack up the truck and head north, she would fall asleep for nearly the entire trip. As soon as we would exit I75 on our way to our campsite, Glace would wake up, stick her head out the window and inhale deeply. She knew where we were and what it meant. She was filled with anticipation and excitement and it was contagious.

One year, we went camping with some friends, who also had a dog. We were going canoeing down the AuSable River and decided to leave the dogs behind. None of us wanted to get tipped out of a canoe into the cold river by an excited dog. It was a quiet trip at the beginning. I had my fishing pole and was casting into deep corners of the river to try and catch some smallmouth bass. I heard a whimper and immediately made everyone stop paddling. I heard it again and realized it was coming from the shore, which was actually a steep, tree-covered embankment. Then I heard the bark and knew there was a dog in trouble in the bushes on the embankment.

My compassion took over. I was ready to jump out of the canoe to find the dog, much to my husband's dismay. As he went over the logistics of getting the canoe to the bank of the river, the dog appeared out of the bushes. I saw the giant head of a chocolate lab. I told the dog to hold on because we were coming, but he paid no attention to my words. He jumped into the icy cold river and swam right to me. The tricky part was getting the dog into the canoe. He was wet, cold and thrilled to see me. Wrestling him into the canoe without tipping it or falling into the river was a miraculous feat and soon we were paddling down the river with a dog in the canoe.

I dubbed him Paddles. We ended up keeping him at our campsite for the entire weekend. He had a collar and tags, but we couldn't reach his family. When it came time for us to go home, the owner of the campground took Paddles and assured me he would continue to try and contact the parents. Of course, when I got home I called and checked to see if he was a man of his word. He was, and Paddles was soon reunited with his family.

Paddles was just one of many lost dogs who have found me. They seem to sense my compassion and come to me. I always take care of them and do my best to find their families. About 90 percent of the time, I'm successful. The other 10 percent, I end up taking the dog to the shelter, but not before I put a flea collar on it and say, "The dog has a collar so you have to hold him until his owner shows up". It took the Animal Control officer in my hometown less than a minute to figure out what I was doing, but he was kind hearted and followed the rule.

Making My Love My Career

In 1994, I founded Special Pet Care Services. Pet Sitting, as an industry, was in its infancy and so was the Internet. So, I trudged off to the library to research what was required to start a business. I checked out a book written by Patti Moran, president of Pet Sitters International. I read the book cover to cover at least four times before I returned it to the library. I took copious notes and found a local insurance agency to write a policy for my business. I ordered business cards, shirts, and pens. I hired an attorney to draft a contract. I got a business phone and a pager and went to work.

I had my first client within a week. My new client was named Ben and he was an elderly Golden Retriever with a kind soul, gentle eyes, and a warm smile. He was also terrified of thunderstorms and would hide behind the hot water heater in the basement. Ben was so frightened if a storm hit it took an hour to get him calm, even with pharmaceutical intervention. Ben's mom was satisfied with my service, so she recommended me to a few of her friends, who also became clients. Those friends recommended me to a few of their friends, and my business started to grow.

This circle of older widows were enjoying their lives and on the go. There were days when they would all go out together, and I took care of eight dogs at one time. I had no idea the 14-15 hours days that lay ahead of me, doing 14-16 visits per day on my own. But at the time, I was happy to be working and making a success out of my business. I had 100% support from Tony and Cyle, but my extended family wasn't as supportive. They gave me a hard time if I missed a family event or was late because I had to work. Eventually, they grew accustomed to me showing for only a few hours and then be off "to do the dogs".

After about four years of strictly pet sitting, I decided to broaden my services to include daily dog walking services. Once I figured out the logistics of the new service, I wondered why I hadn't thought of it sooner. It wasn't long before it was the bread and butter of my business.

My first dog walking clients were a pair of yellow Labrador puppies, Hogan and Reese. They were eight weeks old when I became their dog walker. We spent every lunch hour together. I taught them how to walk on a leash, find treats in a leaf pile, play hide and seek and how to swim in a pool. They loved the pool. We spent five years together before they moved away. I was heartbroken when I found out they were moving out of my service area.

I also got hired by a little Chihuahua/Terrier mix named Mandy. When Cyle would visit with me, Mandy would play King of the Mountain on his back with him lying on the floor. Mandy's mom doted on Cyle and had given me permission for him to visit Mandy. It was a pleasant surprise to realize my clients considered me family, as well as my son and my husband. Cyle has several self-appointed grandmothers, while Tony and I have several other Moms in our lives. Mandy's mom was also the first client who allowed her pet to appear with me in a newspaper article. Once it hit the papers the calls really started rolling in. Mandy's mom retired after about four years of me being her dog walker, but we still stay in touch.

Soon, I was hired to walk a pair of eight-month-old yellow labs who were brothers. Comet and Dozer became the highlight of my day. They were big with square heads and silky golden fur that sparkled in the sunlight. I had been pet sitting/dog walking about eight years when I got hired by their parents. I really bonded with these two boys and our internal clocks synchronized quickly. Soon, they were waiting at the door before I pulled in the driveway. Dozer always met me with a stuffed animal in his mouth and Comet would bounce on his front paws as he barked at me. Each day was the same. Their mom left a snack in the fridge (usually leftovers from dinner the night before, salmon being their favorite). I taught the boys to sit and made sure they did before I dished up their snack. Then, we'd head out for a nice long walk. This routine went on for eight years, on and off. Those dogs didn't know what life was like without me.

I had several other clients who hired me when they got puppies and I loved being part of their whole lives. However, after I had been pet sitting for about a decade I discovered a sorrowful side to the business. Dogs pass away. Since I had garnered so many puppy clients at the beginning of my career, it seemed like they all passed away at the same time. Some of those clients got new puppies, some didn't. Being a part of a dog's whole life as their pet sitter or dog walker is a gift, but it's a gift that comes with pain.

In the middle of a hot summer, I was scheduled to visit a tripod dog named Lena. She had been in my care for several years and I loved her. She had no idea she was challenged and was a very happy dog. This particular trip, her parents were going to separate cities and when I made my first visit, they were both on planes headed in opposite directions. When I walked in, I found Lena on the kitchen floor. I thought she was sleeping. As I approached her, I realized she wasn't sleeping. Alarm bells rang in my head. I fell to my knees to check her and realized she had vomited on the floor and voided her bladder. She was panting heavily and her stomach was bloated. She couldn't get up. Her gums were pale and her eyelids were almost white.

This was serious. I tried to call both of her parents to no avail. I knew it would be hours before I could actually get in touch with them, so I loaded her up in my car and raced to the emergency veterinarian. They knew I was coming and met me with a sling so we could carry her into the clinic. We made it to the exam room and the vet was in the room immediately. Lena's blood pressure was dropping and the vet suspected her spleen was bleeding, so they took her in for an x-ray. Her spleen had ruptured from a tumor and she was bleeding out. The vet believed she had been in pain for some time and we both wondered how her parents had missed it. I imagined that Lena hid it well from them and waited for me as to not burden her parents.

Once the vet made the diagnosis, a decision to put her out of her misery had to be made. We made phone call after phone call to her parents and it was an hour before we finally got in touch with them and got permission to end her suffering. I was helpless to make this decision for her, despite having a contract signed stating that I could make the decision. The vet wouldn't do it until he had talked to her parents. I stayed by her side until it was over. I held her paw and balled her fur in my fists. I rested my head on her chest as she stopped breathing. I sat with her for another 20 minutes, whispering apologies and regrets into her ear. I made the vet take Lena out of the room so I wasn't leaving her behind when I left the clinic. I remember going home that night and sobbing in the shower.

I couldn't sleep that night and had nightmares about Lena. During the following days, I started having flashbacks about the scene in the kitchen and what happened at the vet's office. It was relentless and I was struggling. I didn't know it at the time, but I was suffering from moral distress. I knew what had to be done, but I was powerless to help Lena without her parent's approval. This ordeal with Lena was the beginning of my battle with compassion fatigue. At the time I had no idea what was happening to me, so I continued to work.

Remember Ben? When he passed away from old age, his mom got a new puppy. Another beautiful Golden Retriever, whom she named "Carol's Own Holly B." Naming her cherished dog after me was the best gift anyone has ever given me. I still get misty when I think about it. We called her Beanie and I was her daily dog walker and pet sitter. We became close and I loved taking care of her. Her ears were so soft when I petted them I could barely feel them. She also loved bread. Every time we'd go on a walk, she would look for bread that someone had left out for the birds.

Most of the time I'd see it first, but every once in a while she would nab it before I saw it, then turn and smile at me.

Soon, Beanie got a new brother named Reilly. A larger Golden Retriever, from the same family as Beanie. He had a big blocky head and a belly made to be rubbed. Together, this was a happy family and I loved taking care of them. Actually, the whole family enjoyed spending time with Beanie and Reilly.

I taught the dogs how to slide down a slide at the local playground. We'd take long walks on the beach together. I bonded as tightly with these two dogs as if they were my own. The time came when Beanie slowed down with age and soon the day came to say goodbye. Her mom was recovering from a shoulder injury and couldn't take Beanie to the veterinarian, so she asked me to do it. Of course, I said yes. Beanie didn't know life without me and I wasn't going to let her cross the rainbow bridge without someone who loved her by her side. I felt it was my obligation to both Beanie and her mom. I loved them both so much.

The transition was difficult for me, which surprised me. Usually, I can hold it together until I get home and in the shower, where I let all of my grief out. But, when I was with Beanie I lost it in the vet's office and had to have some time to myself to pull myself together before I left. Once again, I had to make the vet take the dog's body out of the room before I left so I wouldn't be leaving her behind by leaving the room first. I should have noticed this subtle change in my behavior. I chalked it up to an over attachment to a lovely dog that I didn't own. It wasn't.

By this time, I knew something was amiss. I was more cranky than normal with my family. I was starting to be short with my clients. Still, I persevered and continued to work long hours and days. My 8-hour days turned into 14-15 hour days and I would work seven days a week. Sometimes I worked for several months without a day off. I continued to push myself because if I didn't, I felt useless. The compulsion to continue to work coupled with the exhaustion and nightmares were the elements of a brewing storm. I had no life outside of work, other than Tony and Cyle, and inevitably, if they wanted to spend time with me they would have to go with me to work.

During my time as a professional pet sitter, I have accompanied many pets through the end of life process. I have held many paws while these wonderful companions took their last breaths. Each and every one of them affected me, even if I didn't realize it at the time. Some of these experiences are still too difficult to relive, even in the written form, and I still work to come to terms with them.

A Calling

Along with the pet sitting, I had a drive to answer the call for help for pets during disasters; natural or manmade. From the floods in Missouri in 1993, 9/11, Hurricane Katrina through to Hurricane Sandy, I have been involved in providing relief to animals in need through local donation drives. Being in personal contact with someone at ground zero during these disasters gave me a unique perspective of how animals are affected. And, this too, took its toll on me. The letters from the shelters, the pictures of the animals involved and the stories of the suffering were unbearable, and simultaneously why I had to help.

In the aftermath of Hurricane Katrina, several pet professionals in my area, including me, got together to go to New Orleans and bring back pets that had been abandoned. We ended up with more than a dozen dogs and 20 cats. The trip started with 15 cats, but a momma cat delivered kittens en route to Michigan, so there were five tiny kittens added to our group. My part in the effort was to house five of the dogs at a local kennel and take care of them on a daily basis. I was friends with the kennel owner and she was more than happy to help me out. When the animals arrived in Michigan, they were all in a state of shock. I could see it in their eyes. They had a glazed over look and were too quiet in the crates.

We set up a makeshift assembly line so the animals could be looked at by a local veterinarian, microchipped by the local animal shelter and distributed among the volunteers who were housing them. I was assigned the bigger dogs because the kennel had the most room, so I brought back two labs, two pit bull mixed breeds and one large spaniel. I was advised not to name them and just see to their basic needs. That proved impossible for me and I ended up naming all five of them. Within a week the story had hit the newspaper in our little town and four out of five of my dogs were adopted.

The spaniel was left behind and it broke my heart. He was sweet, attentive and well-mannered. I named him Stormy. I spent an hour, twice a day, at the kennel tending to Stormy. I wanted to bring him home, but Tony had taken a stand and said, "No!" And, he was right to do so. Stormy and I spent our days walking the property of the kennel, chasing tennis balls and bonding. It took nearly six weeks to find Stormy a home, but when we did, I was happy for him. He deserved a good home after everything he had been through.

I had noticed, during my time with him, that I wasn't feeling well. I was experiencing a general lack of energy and other symptoms that weren't normal for me even when I was overtired or overworked. I went to my doctor, who, at first, couldn't find anything wrong. Then, I told him about Stormy. My doctor is a dog person and I pet sat for his dogs, so he loved to hear my stories. Something clicked in his head as I talked about Stormy and he ordered blood work and other tests. A week later, he had a diagnosis. I was suffering from an internal fungal infection brought about by working with the dogs that had been languishing in the dirty water in New Orleans.

I'll just say that the treatment was worse than the infection and, even though I was seriously ill, I continued to work. I felt compelled to work. The images and stories I had heard from Hurricane Katrina stuck with me like glue and I couldn't shake them. I assumed we were all suffering through the same thing, with the graphic images on TV and the reporters doing their best to find the most horrific, heart-wrenching stories to broadcast. But, since my story is the only one I can share with any sort of insight, I hope it helps someone else who is suffering.

When Hurricane Sandy hit, it hit the shores of Lake Huron as well as the shores of the Atlantic. While we didn't sustain the damage seen in New Jersey, we had our share of trouble. Large trees had fallen over many power lines and we were without power for a week. For miles along the shore our beaches had been destroyed. We experienced 20-foot waves on Lake Huron, which is highly unusual. When the waves crashed on our beaches, they left nothing behind. It was devastating.

After Hurricane Sandy, I started a donation drive for The Humane Society of Atlantic County in New Jersey, but something wasn't right with me. I gave this donation drive my all and it proved to be the biggest donation drive I had ever pulled off. It garnered me an Honorable Mention for the Platinum Paw Award with PSI.

I continued to work as a pet sitter and a dog walker, while doubling as the administrator of a huge donation drive. I felt overcome with grief. I knew nothing about compassion fatigue or that it was something one could suffer from. I had no idea that my grief from the past 20 years was accumulating. I assumed that this particular donation drive had gotten the best of me because it had literally hit home.

In addition to my personal grief, I was becoming my town's grief counselor for pets. Clients would count on me to help them through their own grief over losing their pet. Strangers would call and ask my opinion about if it was time to put their pet down because their vet wouldn't give them a straight answer and they needed guidance. People would recognize me in the grocery store or pet store and tell me their stories of grief about their pets. Pets are an equalizer. Pet lovers will talk to a complete stranger if it's about their pet.

One perfectly ordinary day, while walking two of my daily dogs, I started to feel hungry. I was only about one-quarter of the way through the walk and wondered how hungry I would be by the time we got back from our walk and if my sugar would drop. I remember debating whether we should turn around or just keep going because the dogs hadn't pooped yet. I knew they had to poop, but that day they seemed to be taking too much time. I was growing hungry and, frankly, impatient. Then like a termite boring into a piece of wood, the thought came to me, 'These dogs are so selfish'. I cringe when I think about it. I should have paid more attention to this thought because it was out of character for me. We did finish the walk and the dogs finally pooped, but I was none the wiser for my self-centered thought. Something changed in that moment and that thought hung on for quite some time, although I refused to let it have any power.

Instead of introspection, I stubbornly worked even harder. Everything had to be perfect. I couldn't say no to my clients and I isolated myself from my family. I had trouble deciding what to wear, what to eat, which chore to do first. My insomnia became a constant. I couldn't sleep through the night if I was lucky enough to fall asleep at all. I didn't want to talk to anyone other than my dogs.

What I later learned was compassion fatigue tightened its grip on me; I started to become hypersensitive in many ways. If I was around people, I felt like they didn't want me there or that I was a bother. I became intolerant of loud noises which would induce in me a flash of anger. My startle reflex was over-reactive. I also became sensitive to strong smells. Some made me sick, while others seemed to induce a flood of emotions that left me wrung out, especially fresh cut grass. I was easily frightened by strangers using stern voices. I started to become slightly paranoid and was easily insulted.

I began to experience graphic intrusive images. They started with images I was familiar with -- Lena on her kitchen floor, the dogs from Hurricane Katrina, other dogs who had become severely ill on my watch, pets whose paws I held as they took their last breath, the image of my calico cat as she lay dying on couch, Bear, and even as far back as Pansy's dead puppies. These images would flash before me at any time. I could be doing anything like cooking dinner or talking to a client and I would be assaulted by a disturbing image and then it would be gone. I began to question my own stability. Was I overtired? Overworked? Was I not dealing with things? I spoke to my doctor about it and was prescribed antidepressants and anti-anxiety meds. While I will admit they were helpful, they really didn't get to the root of the problem. My doctor wasn't familiar with compassion fatigue and I still didn't know what was wrong with me, so when the meds took the edge of the anxiety. I found relief—for a while.

Waves of Trauma

Things took a bitter turn for me in August of 2013. My father-in-law, who was bravely battling ALS had taken a fall at his home. Tony's step-mother called us to help him get up off the floor. Thinking we just had to help him get into his favorite chair and catch his breath, we went over to his house. My mother-in-law hurried us into the bedroom where we found him face down on the floor. I thought he was in pain and waiting for us to help him up. I shook him to let him know we were there, but he was cold to my touch. I looked at Tony, who was already pale and in the beginning stages of shock, and motioned to him to help me roll his dad over.

When we did, we saw that his dad was unconscious and barely breathing. He was taking shallow gasps and his face was gray. EMS arrived shortly after we did. They revived him and then rushed to the ER where they spent six hours stabilizing him in order to move him to ICU. We spent the next 17 days at the hospital, most of them in the ICU. Machines constantly droned in the background. Sights and smells registered in my subconscious as Tony and I spent as much time as possible with him.

Tony's father passed away on September 3, the day before our 25th wedding anniversary. I was the second person to arrive at the hospital after he died. Most of the family was an hour or more away. My mother-in-law was still with him when I walked in. I stayed with her to wait for the rest of the family and, ultimately, the funeral home. The worst part of this experience was when the funeral home arrived and asked us to escort this once lively, bigger-than-life man down the elevator in a body bag that looked like a blue quilt. I couldn't do it. I had to take the stairs.

Family drama seemed to supersede grief, so my grief was never processed. I just held it in and held it together. I gave myself the luxury of breaking down during the funeral when the Air Force contingent played taps and my nephew, who was active Air Force, folded the flag and presented it to my mother-in-law. I was sobbing so hard I could barely breathe. I held my husband's hand as grief overtook him. That was the extent of our shared grieving. The day after the funeral, we both went back to work as if life was still normal.

I had just endured a tremendous trauma. Now, the intrusive imagery and nightmares were of my father-in-law's gray face when we turned him over or the moment we saw him in the ICU hooked to the ventilator. Since I refused to acknowledge them, the images lingered. Soon, they were accompanied by aromas. The sights and smells that I barely registered in the hospital were rushing back to fuel the nightmares and imagery. I said nothing. Stubbornly refusing to acknowledge them or the grief I was feeling, I continued to work. I felt *compelled* to work, although the work wasn't the same for me. Now, instead of joy being with the dogs, I felt fear.

Four months later, on a cold January day in the dead of a Michigan winter, I got a phone call from Florida saying my mom was going in for a cardiac catheterization. She had undergone a major heart surgery years earlier. I was concerned, but I didn't jump on a plane to Florida to be at her bedside. We didn't have a good relationship and I knew my brother was there to take care of her. Two days later I called the hospital to see how she was doing and the news wasn't good. She wasn't awake or sedated. She was in a coma and had been since the operation.

Ten days later Mom regained consciousness but was completely paralyzed. When I called to talk to her, she refused to speak to me. She was angry and bitter because she had signed a Do Not Resuscitate Order and it had been ignored. My brother had taken over as her healthcare advocate. He was as angry and bitter as Mom and, true to form; he took it out on me. Talking to him in a reasonable manner was impossible. His verbal assault and abuse added to my trauma, but I didn't acknowledge it.

My mother's decline lasted for seven months. She never made it home. Her brain had been deprived of oxygen for several minutes during her surgery. If the DNR had been followed, as she had requested, she wouldn't have had to endure the seven months of paralysis or the seizures that further injured her brain.

I never went to Florida to see Mom because of my brother's bullying. As with all my previous trauma, graphic imagery haunted me. The anxiety and guilt of not going to Florida to say goodbye to my mom were intensified when the imagines from my childhood bullying and violence from my brother started to surface.

What Is Wrong With Me?

We lost 20 pets in the course of six months at this time in my business. I was witness to some (primary trauma), others from the owners rehashing their experiences for me (vicarious trauma). I couldn't find it within myself to comfort them. In fact, I would get angry about owners expecting to find solace from me.

The straw that broke the camel's back arrived in the form of a hospice care situation for one of my long time pet sitting clients. A wonderful, delicate little dog, that I had cared for since she was two, was well into her teens and her time was growing short. Her parents did everything they could to keep her healthy, but the aging process has its own terms. They decided it was time to let her go, and set a date for the following Friday. They called and asked me to make lunchtime visits every day the following week. Hospice visits. Of course, I said yes. The compulsion to work was still stronger than the grief I was feeling.

I went to see this little dog every day that week knowing in the back of my mind that she had an appointment to end her life. I couldn't take it. I cried at every visit. I thought about canceling the assignment. I wondered if I could actually call in sick. Then, I found myself hoping I wouldn't wake up in the morning. I had no intention of inflicting self-harm, but the thought of not waking up in the morning kept recurring. The nightmares continued — graphic, apocalyptic, intense and frightening — leaving me depleted and rattled when I woke up. I was starting to acknowledge the tremendous weight of my grief. I felt completely useless.

I knew I was in big trouble. One day, I sat down with a cup of coffee and a journal on my back deck. I thought about what was happening to me. Was I becoming mentally unstable? Did I need professional help? Was I simply overwhelmed and overworked? It was time to be brutally honest with myself about what I was thinking and feeling and my lack of control over my thoughts. I put pen to paper expecting to write a novel, but the only thing I wrote down that day was, "My heart isn't in it anymore because my heart is broken."

I had lived with this pain for years before I sat down with that journal. Still, I had no clarity about what was wrong, what "it" was. I felt frightened and overwhelmed, so I grabbed at a chance to run. My husband had been offered a job with Boeing and it was the perfect excuse to get away from "it". I handed over my business to my business manager, packed my house and my family and moved to Seattle.

Initially, it seemed to help. I felt better because I wasn't working and I was busy with unpacking and getting settled. But, that was only on the surface. I couldn't run away from my brain. The intrusive thoughts still came at all hours of the day. The nightmares continued. I was hypervigilant. Tony was working which gave me the perfect excuse to further isolate. My brain started to feel like an enemy. How do you wage war on your own brain? You don't. You can't. Instead, you pay attention to what your brain is doing and listen to what it's trying to tell you. It was trying to get my attention.

In hindsight, had we not moved to Seattle, I don't know where I would be today. Moving to Seattle afforded me the opportunity to stop moving deeper into compassion fatigue and be still enough to recover and rest. Had I stayed in Michigan, I can assure you this would not have happened.

"It" Has a Name

My epiphany came on an ordinary day. While perusing Facebook, I found an article about Dr. Sophia Yin on a friend's page. I loved Dr. Yin. She was a pioneer in positive reinforcement training with dogs and I had read her book. I had watched her training episodes on YouTube. A happier, more in touch trainer would have been hard to find, in my mind. I recalled that she had taken her own life, but this article explained WHY. As I started to read the article, I saw myself in it.

"It" finally had a name: Compassion Fatigue. The word fatigue doesn't cover the severity of this condition. Fatigue seems to insinuate that you can rest and recover. This is far from true. As I dug further into the research, I realized that compassion fatigue is prevalent in the animal care industry. It's just not discussed.

Compassion Fatigue is a byproduct of caring and all caregivers are susceptible to it. Jessica Dolce describes it as a natural consequence of what we do. It stems from the physical and emotional exhaustion that comes from the constant demand of caring, and from the interaction with the animals we are helping and caring for.

Additionally, we, as pet sitters, care for both our client's pets and our clients. Because we care, we are vulnerable to compassion fatigue. We are also susceptible to burnout which results from the stresses that arise from our work environment. As a matter of fact, Dr. Bernard Rollin, Ph.D. author of the paper "Euthanasia, Moral Stress, and Chronic Illness in Veterinary Medicine" believes that, as pet sitters, we are more vulnerable to compassion fatigue than veterinarians and shelter workers because we straddle both worlds of caring for animals and caring for people. It is inevitable that somewhere along the line in your career as a pet sitter, you will suffer from compassion fatigue.

It is a gradual erosion of what makes us compassionate. The qualities that make us exceptional in our profession also make us susceptible. It is not a disease or a mental illness, but a set of symptoms that manifest differently in different people. If you are experiencing compassion fatigue you will probably recognize some of the classic symptoms. Jessica Dolce's list of symptoms include:

1. Bone Tired Exhaustion. For me, it was the feeling of being so tired that the thought of putting pants on made me wince. Sweatpants or yoga pants became my standard outfit and I'd put pajamas on as soon as I got home from walking dogs or doing pet sitting rounds.

2. Disconnection. I was unable to center or ground myself. It felt as if my brain wasn't attached to my body and the signals weren't being interpreted correctly. I was tripping and even falling often. I wasn't able to be fully present.

3. Sleeping difficulties. I suffered from not being able to fall asleep and not being able to stay asleep. For some, the difficulty is in sleeping too much.

4. Persistent Physical Ailments. I had stomach issues, headaches, grinding of my teeth, a lump in my throat, joint pain, muscle aches, fatigue, and ringing in my ears.

5. Anger or irritability. I was angry about things that would not have bothered me in the past. For example, I found myself angry with a dog in my care for peeing on the rug and resenting that I had to clean it up.

6. Nightmares and flashbacks. I had graphic nightmares and flashbacks that took me back to the moments of a trauma over and over again.

7. Difficulty concentrating and forgetfulness. I would read a passage in a book four or five times and finally realize I had already read it. I forgot appointments, lost keys, and other items.

8. Cynicism. Eye-rolling is a trigger signal for me. When I start rolling my eyes, I know I'm backsliding. Previously, I would be grateful and excited when a client wanted to get a new pet, instead, I was dreading how my burden was multiplied. _My entire world view had changed_. This is extremely important as a symptom of compassion fatigue as opposed to burnout.

9. Hypervigilance. I was always alert for the bad guy in the bushes and my flight or fight response was "on" all of the time.

10. Exaggerated Startle Response. Things that wouldn't usually startle me now scared the wits out of me. My husband sneaking up behind me to poke me in the ribs nearly cost him a broken nose as I immediately balled my hand into a fist to throw a punch. A slamming door would send me into tears.

11. Isolation From Others. I withdrew from pleasurable activities, people, relationships, in fact, everything that wasn't work. When I couldn't completely isolate, I distanced myself by staying busy.

12. Intrusive Imagery. I was assaulted by imagery at all times and places. There was no defense against these intrusions. For example, I was walking on a quiet path in the woods enjoying the fresh air, warm sun and the birds

twittering away in the trees beyond. Suddenly, I would see a picture in my head of a beaten and abused dog I assisted the week before. I was overtaken by grief. THAT is intrusive imagery and I found it to be one of the most distressing parts of compassion fatigue.

13. No Life Outside Of Work. I've used every excuse there is like, "Who has time?" or "The only friends I have are at work", or even "I have no interest in life outside of work". While these may be symptoms of a workaholic, they very well may be a symptom of compassion fatigue, especially if this isn't normal for you.

14. Reduced Ability To Feel Sympathy Or Empathy. It is frightening when the very things that make pet sitters great at their jobs are falling away. A perfect example is a shelter worker who, instead of telling herself that the old lady who just dropped her dog off at the shelter is probably feeling guilty or sad, judges the lady harshly and may even post a derogatory comment on social media about this heartless old lady. If you find yourself judging the actions of others harshly, especially those actions involving their pets, self-introspection is strongly advised. Additionally, if you find yourself losing your sympathy for a client who just lost their pet, it's time to dig deep and assess your situation.

15. Heightened Arousal Response. I hate discord. Yet, during the depths of compassion fatigue, I would get confrontational instead of backing down. A perfect example of this happened one day when I was in a PetSmart parking lot. As I got out of my car, I noticed someone had left their dog in their car with the windows cracked just a bit. I had been on a kick that summer about leaving dogs in hot cars and was *immediately* furious. There was no simmering. I went from calm to furious in a flash. I stormed into the store and demanded that the manager either call this person out or call the Sheriff. Keep in mind that all of the employees in this store knew me and they also knew this was not normal behavior for me. The manager refused to pursue any action, so I stormed out of the store, found a rock and intended to break the window of this person's car. I wasn't thinking at all. I was just a roiling mass of fury. Fortunately for me, someone else had found this dog and had already called the Sheriff who was in the process of breaking the window himself.

16. Suicidal Thoughts or Actions. Thoughts of self-harm are an obvious sign, but more insidious are the thoughts that don't involve self-harm, such as, "I hope I don't wake up tomorrow". While this may seem like a passing thought, it

is actually a red flag to seek help and quickly. Risky behavior that could result in death, such as not buckling a seat belt and hoping to get into an accident is a Red Flag! If you are having these thoughts, please call The National Suicide Prevention Hotline right now. 1-800-273-TALK. Put the book down right now and call.

These are some of the most common symptoms of compassion fatigue. Different people experience symptoms in different ways. The point is that the person is suffering from an occupational hazard that ebbs and flows. Some experts believe that once you've experienced compassion fatigue you are likely to experience it again. Others believe you can recover completely. The one thing experts do agree on is that it is real and it distorts one's world view.

There are four factors that contribute to compassion fatigue and its progression. You can experience just one or experience all four of them.

1. Primary Trauma. These are situations that put you directly on the front line. This includes direct grief situations over which you have no control. In this situation, you have directly experienced the trauma, whether it be the death of a loved one or watching a horrific incident. Anything that you witness first-hand

that causes an intense reaction can be considered trauma. The size of the trauma doesn't matter. Your reaction does. Example: Let's say you have accidentally hit and killed a dog on your way to a client's home. I know, it's awful, but stay with me. This is an example of primary trauma.

2. Secondary Trauma. You are not in direct danger, but you are bearing witness to the suffering of others. You could be listening to someone's trauma or retelling your own traumatic story. Either way, you are bearing witness to the suffering of others. Even watching videos online can be secondary trauma if they affect you. Continuing to use our example, you saw another car accidentally hit and kill the dog while driving to a client's home. You saw the trauma and witnessed the dog's suffering and/or the other driver's suffering. If you stop to talk to the person who hit the dog, you will be experiencing secondary trauma by listening to that person tell their story.

3. Vicarious Trauma. This is a direct result of bearing witness to trauma, whether it's primary or secondary. You are not in harm's way, but you are vicariously witnessing the

trauma; such as you have a reaction to a story you've been told by another pet care professional that may not have experienced the trauma but still had a strong reaction to it. In our example, this would manifest as your client saw the dog accidentally get hit and killed. She then proceeded to tell you about it once you arrived at her home. Her reaction is intense and disturbing, and in turn, so is yours.

4. PTSD. While primarily a diagnoses for soldiers who have experienced the violence and disturbing images of war, PTSD is the anxiety associated with trauma. The anxiety of PTSD is intense and life altering. Using the same example, PTSD would manifest as severe anxiety as you drive because of your experience with hitting and killing the dog, whether it was a primary, secondary or vicarious trauma. The situation has altered your worldview and produced anxiety that alters the way you live your life.

As you read through this book, you will be experiencing vicarious trauma. Any reaction on your part to any of the stories is considered vicarious trauma. While writing this book, I experienced secondary trauma because I was reliving the traumas as I wrote about them. This is how compassion fatigue sneaks up on you. If you've been affected by any of the stories you've read so far, make a note of it. Write down what your reaction was and how you felt about it. Please acknowledge it.

Many people mistake compassion fatigue for burnout. While they may share a few signs and symptoms, they are not the same thing.

Burnout stems from the environment in which you work. "It derives its frustration from your low job satisfaction. It builds up over time due to excessive and prolonged stress from your job." *Jessica Dolce*. A vacation may help alleviate the symptoms of burnout. It's temporary and the world outside of your job doesn't adversely affect you. Burnout does not affect your world view. It leaves you cranky, tired and less than enthusiastic about your job. A key component of compassion fatigue is the compulsion to work. If you're suffering from burnout, staying in bed all day is appealing. If you're suffering from compassion fatigue, while staying in bed seems appealing, you are compelled to get out of bed and go do your job.

Once I realized the difference between compassion fatigue and burnout I realized I was experiencing many of the symptoms of compassion fatigue as well as PTSD.

You Have to Crawl Before Walking

The most devastating part of compassion fatigue, for me, was it robbed me of one of my biggest joys as a pet sitter. My sparkle with animals was gone. The loss of my compassion for animals rendered me practically useless as a pet sitter and distressed me greatly.

For the first time in my life, after we moved to Seattle, I took a break from working and pushing myself. I took a break from being a perfectionist. I gave myself permission to sleep in, to take adventures, to eat better, to stop punishing myself and to just "be" with myself. This took a tremendous effort on my part, but it was essential.

I found resources online to help me battle compassion fatigue. The most helpful was Jessica Dolce's eight-week online course, Compassion In Balance. Jessica is a fellow pet care professional who works with rescue groups and shelters. Not only has she suffered from compassion fatigue, she has witnessed what compassion fatigue has done to the people around her. She knows her stuff and was insightful and helpful throughout my recovery process.

Through taking this course, I learned about what triggers stress and distress in me. I learned what to do with the graphic imagines and intrusive thoughts. I knew what to do about the nightmares and I started to get my power back over the traumas I had endured. By the end of it, I had my own personalized workbook on how to deal with compassion fatigue, stress, anxiety, trauma, and PTSD.

While taking this course, I had a clash with a bully. He lived in the condo below us and one day our dogs had a run-in. No harm came to either dog, but the bully used it as fodder for his actions towards my dogs and me. He bullied my dogs, me and other residents. The bully would scream obscenities at my dogs and at me through open windows in our condo if the dogs were running around. If he thought I was making too much noise, he would pound on his ceiling until I stopped whatever I was doing. I felt I had to sit still and hide in my own home. My hypervigilance kicked in and I lived in a state of heightened anxiety for months.

He was loud, angry and menacing. He threatened my dogs repeatedly, which made me so fearful I quit my part time job to stay home and protect them. The list of his aggressions was long and ongoing. I took as much legal action as possible to keep myself safe from him, but there was only so much I could do. I lived in fear until we moved out.

I know this situation slowed my recovery, but it did not stop it. I maintained forward motion. I knew I was getting better because I wasn't confronting him. If it had happened the summer before, I know there would have been a physical encounter because I had no control over my arousal response.

I continued to put things in perspective and I used the tools that I was learning in Jessica's course. I found that most days I was okay -- not great, but okay. However, when I started to think about throwing eggs at the bully's head, I knew I was moving in the wrong direction. Being bullied takes your power, and while this has little to do with compassion fatigue, it does cause a regression of symptoms. I gained this perspective through taking Jessica Dolce's course

Recovery was and is a long process filled with hard work, small joys and self-introspection. It took dedicated effort and I couldn't have made it without my personalized workbook and the support of my husband. I battled some monsters and finally took them down. I faced some character flaws about myself and figured out how to make them useful. I took this endeavor seriously. I left no stone unturned. I was surprised at how much research has been done in the animal care world but was flummoxed that no research had been done specifically for pet sitters. Despite that fact, I took what I needed from the research available for others in the Pet Care Industry.

While I continue to recover from compassion fatigue, I'm not the same person I was a year ago. I'm more self-aware, I listen to the thoughts in my head and, when they turn negative, I challenge them and get out my personalized workbook. I don't overwork myself, I rest when I'm tired, eat when I'm hungry and have found some compassion for myself. Recovery is not always a comfortable task, nor is it easy. It's like putting my pants on; some days I just don't want to.

Despite my setbacks, my compassion came back, slowly and cautiously, like a shy kitten who isn't sure if you are going to hurt it or pet it. I am patient and let the compassion return in its own time. It is a process and recovery cannot be rushed. I couldn't make a list, check off the chores accomplished and then say "I'm done!" It doesn't work that way.

Tools

Recovery from compassion fatigue requires a delicate balance of self-care and resiliency-building. In fact, building your resiliency not only helps you recover from compassion fatigue, it's a preventative step you can take before compassion fatigue becomes an issue. Being resilient doesn't make us impervious to stress, distress, trauma or compassion fatigue. But, it will help you recover faster, and your battle with compassion fatigue may be considerably less debilitating. Resiliency allows you to experience the negative emotions of an event without becoming overwhelmed, and to move forward.

When I think of the word resilient, I picture Silly Putty. Do you remember that stuff? You could make it flat on a cartoon and it would pick up the image. You could roll it into a ball and make it bounce. Consider the definition of resilience: "The ability to recover quickly from misfortune; to be able to return to original form after being bent, compressed or stretched out of shape." Silly Putty fits that definition perfectly. In a human, it is the ability to recover quickly from disruptive change or misfortune without being overwhelmed or acting in dysfunctional or harmful ways.

As a pet sitter, resiliency is a required tool. We must have this tool in order to bounce back from adversity because, if we don't, the result is feelings of helplessness, depression, anxiety, shameful defeat and even suicidal thoughts and actions. On the bright side, resiliency can be learned. If you are in any stage of trauma right now, you can take these tools and help yourself recover. It's best if you have some kind of support, a trusted person to talk to, but if you're anything like me, you'll want to do it alone. Please don't. It is so much easier if you let someone help you. Allow someone you trust the privilege of helping you.

Are you ready to become Silly Putty resilient?

1. Eliminate Perfectionism. I can hear you saying "What???" from here! Yep, eliminate it! Perfectionism is associated with anxiety, helplessness, and shameful defeat and can lead to suicidal thoughts and actions, so why not eliminate it?

Consider the Japanese tradition of Wabi-sabi. Each tea cup is handmade and thereby imperfect, but still useful. As the teacup is chipped and cracked from use, the chips and cracks are filled in with gold. The once imperfect tea cup, with time and use, has become priceless. Now, imagine your chips and cracks are filled with gold instead of guilt. How priceless are you? Holding on to perfection disconnects us from appreciating our mistakes and filling them with gold.

2. Let Go of Control. Again, I can hear you groan. Being the "General Manager of Everything" is exhausting, but you do it because....? I can answer that for you. You do it because no one else can do it as well as you can. Right? It's okay to admit that. I used to be a control monster. My control needs went beyond control freak straight into control monster. I had to learn to let go of control. Start with small things. Consider Silly Putty. You can control the shape you form it into. You can influence the Silly Putty's trajectory when you toss it, but you can't control its bounce. When you start to let go of things and delegate tasks to other people, think of the Japanese tradition of Wabi-sabi and fill their cracks and chips with gold. Be realistic about what you actually can control which is little, what you are able to influence, which is a bit more, and what is actually outside of your control which is most things.

3. Find Meaning in your Work. Since you are reading the book, I assume that you are suffering in some way and have lost your connection to your work. You are getting up, doing your job, but have lost touch with the passion you once had for what you are doing. In order to reconnect with your work, ask yourself, "Have I done good work today?" Are you continuing to move, however incrementally, toward your goals? What would make you feel you have helped today? Is there even a moment or small action that would give meaning to your work today? Ponder these questions as you think about your connection to your work. As you reconnect to the meaning in your work, you will build resiliency. You will be able to feel the negative emotions of an incident, yet be able to move forward. Like Silly Putty, you will be able to bounce back.

4. Reframe Your Problem. This requires a change of perspective on your part and probably a change in attitude. Consider it a challenge instead of a threat to look at a problem from a different angle. Find a way to reconstruct the problem which will open the way for more creative solutions. Don't label. Reframe! Instead of thinking your client is being difficult for calling four times in one day; consider WHY your client feels the need to call you four times in one day. Are you not meeting his need the first time he calls? Is there a different way to meet that need? Are there outside factors that may be influencing him to call four times? Reshape your Silly Putty and bounce.

5. Be Kind to Yourself. If your friend or family member were suffering from the very thing you are suffering from, what would you do? Apply Wabi-sabi to yourself. Are you cracking and chipping yourself unnecessarily? Instead, take the time to fill in the cracks and chips with gold. Be kind to yourself. Challenge your negative self-talk. Identify that voice in your head and challenge it. Is it a parent? A teacher? Find and physically hang out with kind people. Treat yourself like a friend.

6. Be Part of Something Greater. This applies to both your work and your life outside of work. Outside of work could be anything from a church to a book club. It's bigger than you and you can contribute to it. The challenge here is your work life. Pet sitters, by nature, spend much of their time alone. It's very easy to disconnect and feel isolated. In order to connect to something greater in your professional life, consider joining a professional organization specifically for pet sitters. Imagine that you are connected with all of the other pet sitters in the world. We all have a connection to each other simply based on the work that we do. If you are still struggling with this, it's okay. You may not be ready.

When I got to this stage, I ended up going to local dogs parks, on my own, to just sit and watch the dogs play. I met many kind people, who, although they didn't know my situation, were kind and caring towards me just because they knew I was a dog lover. Using the fact that I was a dog lover was social glue that allowed me to connect with people I didn't know. They didn't judge me or add to my suffering. They allowed me to love on their dogs, to have polite conversations with like-minded people and, if I was lucky, to give their dog a treat or throw a ball for them. Eventually, I ended up volunteering my time at cleanups at this dog park simply because I felt that the dog park was something bigger than me and I was part of it. It was a small and healing step for me.

Take our Silly Putty example. You can add two or three other clumps of Silly Putty to make a huge Silly Putty ball that will bounce with a much greater velocity than if you only used only one. The people and animals and even the dog park became other clumps of Silly Putty for me.

7. Accept and Embrace Change. If someone had told me in early 2015 that I would have to accept and embrace change, I would have fallen over laughing. I had lived and worked in the same small town in Michigan my entire life. The only change I had to deal with was moving to a new house and I only did that three times. Now, a year later, I live 2000 miles away from that small town, in a different time zone, in a different climate, in a different home, in Seattle. How did I manage this? I had to accept and embrace the change. It wasn't easy and some days it's still a challenge. But, here I am. While I certainly don't expect that you will have to move 2000 miles in order to accept and embrace change, there are changes you can make and accept gracefully.

First, appreciate the ways your body is going to change as you age. I know it stinks, but it happens and even if you have a plastic surgeon on speed dial, nature has its own agenda. Changes can be difficult, sometimes startling, sometimes pleasant, and take some time to accept. Changes are often even more difficult to embrace. Apply Wabi-sabi and see how that affects your perception of these changes. (I don't know how a hot flash can be filled with gold, but I'm trying).

Second, acknowledge the losses in your life. This step is the most difficult as I tend to stuff my grief. But, in order to bounce, I had to acknowledge the losses and the feelings of grief in order to move forward. You may want to write your feelings down in a journal, use balloons to let them go, or seek professional help if you need it. Give your feelings respect and reverence. It does not matter if someone agrees with or understands your grief. You are feeling it and you have to acknowledge it. Acknowledging and allowing yourself to feel your grief doesn't make its impact on your compassion fatigue worse. Instead, it takes away the power of your grief to build up and lay you flat.

Third, understand that surprises will happen along the way. Good ones, bad ones and sometimes, extraordinary ones. You can prepare for surprises by building your resiliency and by working on the things I've just suggested. The one constant in life is change.

Pollyanna had it right when she looked for the good in every situation. She gets a bad rap, by the way. Look for the good in a situation, instead of the bad. Use Wabi-sabi.

7. Practice Self-Care. In addition to building resiliency, you must learn and practice self-care. Dr. Figley and Dr. Rollin, both Ph.D. professors working in the field of compassion fatigue, agree that, as pet sitters, we are in a unique situation in the pet care industry. We are often privy to certain aspects of a client's life that a veterinarian would not usually be included in. We spend time in the homes and lives of our clients and it is easy to get too involved. We need to be careful about what we allow into our personal lives when it comes to our clients. This creates an environment for moral stress and distress that can lead us further down the path of compassion fatigue. It is why self-care is so important.

We are also faced with the killing/caring paradox in our industry. The pet care industry (including veterinarians, shelter workers and vet techs) is the ONLY industry where we are tasked with making end-of-life decisions concerning the lives we provide care for. This paradox induces primary and secondary trauma, as well as moral distress. We are faced with an ethical quandary because we have to act in a manner that may be contrary to our personal or professional values, thus causing moral distress. In addition, we are given no time to process our emotions and are always in a cycle of grief.

Self-care is crucial and essential to recover from compassion fatigue. There are dozens of books and articles about how each of these will contribute to one's sense of well-being and it's difficult to know which is best. I believe that there isn't just one way to take care of yourself. Everyone is different, but these five elements are universal: Nutrition, Exercise, Sleep, Self-awareness, Friends & Family. All are easily monitored, although not easily controlled. Addressing these areas is the beginning of self-care.

Nutrition - Scientists are beginning to understand that stress eating is actually a way in which the brain tries to provide comfort the body during times of high stress and anxiety. Perhaps you lose your appetite during times of stress. The food you eat is your fuel. During times of stress, your brain will tell you to go for the highly palatable foods, usually high in carbs, sugar, and fat. Why? Because the carbs, sugar and fat release chemicals in your brain that soothe your anxiety.

During time of stress I cut my carbs, sugar and fat in half and add foods that give me better fuel for my body.

Try cutting back on caffeine and alcohol as well. I know, I know. When given this advice I was hesitant, if not downright stubborn, about it. I'm not a stress eater. I can't eat when I'm stressed or anxious, but I still need to fuel my body. I was living on coffee and No Bake Cookies because I couldn't stomach anything else without getting sick.

Slowly, I replaced the coffee with water and lots of it. I started to eat less No Bakes and started eating bland foods including plain rice, pasta, applesauce, and potatoes. I couldn't eat anything else. I also added a multivitamin to my diet, which helped tremendously. However, if you are a stress eater, your brain is already telling you to eat rice, pasta and potatoes. So, eat them, but only eat half of what you would normally eat to see if that placates your brain and lowers your stress and anxiety.

Pay attention to what happens to your body when your brain tells you to stress eat. Keep a food diary; not for self-judgment but as a way to experiment with the food you eat. And, above all, be kind to yourself. Don't berate yourself. Be an observer of your habits.

Exercise - If you are like me, getting exercise sounds redundant. I walk dogs for over seven miles every day. Do I really need more exercise? Turns out, my heart and lungs do. It's also the last thing I want to do during times of stress. When I was suffering from compassion fatigue, I didn't want to move off of the couch after I got home from walking dogs all day. I was too tired.

I needed to really dig deep for willingness to do this and my heart and my lungs are glad I made the effort. During times of stress, our brain sends corticosteroids into our system to enable flight or fight. Like medicinal steroids, these chemicals will help us run fast if we choose the flight reflex or fight like mad if we choose the fight reflex. These chemicals are helpful and important, but, under chronic stress and anxiety, such as experienced during compassion fatigue, these chemicals stay in our body.

Even if we walk dogs for seven miles, our heart and lungs are still ready for the flight or fight. Those chemicals build up and can cause illness such as hardening of the arteries. I've found a great way to relieve the pressure is to do at least 10 minutes of heart-pounding cardio a day. Ugh, right? The picture that comes to my mind is running and I look like a flamingo when I run. I feel awkward. Going to the gym was out for many reasons, which (in my mind) were valid. Whatever I chose to do, I had to be able to wear my sweat pants and a t-shirt, not have to buy special equipment and not have to be seen in public.

Jessica offered up a Yoga challenge. Do 30 days of Yoga, at my pace in the comfort of my own home. Well, why not? Turns out Yoga is hard work and was just what I needed to help offset the chemicals in my body that were signaling my flight or fight response. My body thanked me. My Doctor even noticed a difference!

Let me stress that your exercise of choice must be something you enjoy doing. Forced exercise releases those pesky stress hormones in your brain, thus rendering forced or coerced exercise futile when it comes to recovering from compassion fatigue. This not the time to buy an expensive gym membership and hire a trainer to push you or force you to work out or engage in exercises that you do not enjoy. You may need to try a few different things to find what works for you.

Sleep - We all know that we need to sleep in order to restore our bodies and minds. But if your sleep is interrupted, chances are your body isn't being restored and your mind is working overtime. Naps, to me, were a waste of time. I couldn't fall asleep easily and I rarely slept through the night. During my battle with compassion fatigue, I was overtaken with nightmares, thus rendering me sleepless for days on end. Who wants to go to sleep to be assaulted by graphic nightmares? So the cycle went. No sleep led to more stress and anxiety which led to less food and more fatigue.

Scientist's opinions vary on how much sleep a body needs to heal and restore energy. Let's say your body needs six hours of restorative sleep. Let's also assume you aren't getting that six hours of sleep because of stress and anxiety. What do you do? Well, you could consult with your doctor, which I recommend, especially if you think you are suffering from compassion fatigue. My doctor wasn't familiar with compassion fatigue, but he trusted me enough as an informed patient that my failure to sleep was because of the stress and anxiety of compassion fatigue.

I received some medicinal aid for sleeping, but I still needed to fight the nightmares. I found that if I awoke during a nightmare and wrote it down, I could go back to sleep — once I turned my pillow over (because my grandma told me this will bury the bad dream). I began to pay attention to my breathing as I lay in bed when I was unable to go to sleep. I found I was barely breathing. Short, small gasps of air were the norm. I began to practice belly breathing so my body would relax, even though was hard for me to focus. My brain would wander to other things and I would return to gasping.

Compassion fatigue steals your ability to concentrate, so the belly breathing activity helped me relax and retrain my brain to focus. It's really easy to do. To start, I had to actually have my hand on my belly to keep me centered. I had to learn to draw a breath in with my belly. Watch a sleeping baby breathe. They use their bellies, not their chests. That's the goal.

Tonight when you go to bed, lie on your back and put your hand on your belly. When you draw a breath in, make sure you hand goes up with your belly. Draw in a big breath to a slow count of 3. Exhale, slowly making sure you hand goes down with your belly to a slow count of 6. You may run out of air before you get to 6 but continue to exhale. Repeat this process, focusing on your hand and your counting. See what happens. You may not fall asleep right away, but you will find that your brain is slowing down and not running down those bunny trails that keep you awake. Try this for 30 nights and see if it helps with your sleeping.

If you wake up with a nightmare, grab a pen and a notepad (I recommend keeping these close to your bed) and write them down, thus releasing their power. Turn your pillow over, and begin your breathing again. Experiment with what works best for you. Most importantly, if you find that you need a nap in the middle of the day—take it! I've learned the value of a power nap.

Another tool to help you relax into sleep is meditation. I recommend iRest meditation. There are several CDs available to help you learn to meditate yourself to sleep.

Self-awareness - Mindfulness. Pay attention to your self-talk. Notice what words you are using and the tone. I would bet you a nickel that it's negative. While battling compassion fatigue, your brain will tell you that you aren't working hard enough or you aren't doing a good job, while pushing you to continue to work. It's distressing! Take the time to be mindful of what you are saying to yourself and challenge it. Instead of being hard on yourself because of your critical self-talk, take a stand and challenge it. This will help your brain refocus on positive things and help you combat your compassion fatigue. It's not easy, though. Habits and patterns are difficult to break and didn't develop overnight. Changing your focus to balance the critical self-talk with positive attributes takes time and continuous effort.

If you are stuck for positive thoughts, find the old notes and cards from your clients that are uplifting and edifying and read them. Notice your reaction. Are you dismissing the positive accolades with a wave of your hand and saying things like, "That wasn't anything special" or "The client is just saying that". I bet you are. I did.

Before becoming more self-aware and listening to the self-talk, I had no idea how much damage I was doing to myself. Becoming mindful of your self-talk is hard work and even the act of being mindful will be met with negativity from your inner voice. Trust me, I know. I said things to myself like, "Oh, I don't need to do that", "I don't have time for this", "This is stupid". However, it is essential that you listen to your self-talk.

Replace the negative with a positive. I had to start small, really small. Instead of saying, "I'm not doing a good job", I had to say, "I'm okay." That tiny shift in my self-talk started to change my perspective and how I treated myself. Adopt a positive mantra about yourself: "I am good enough", "I am a good pet sitter". As you notice the negative self-talk and begin to challenge it, these positive mantras will help you stay the course.

Additionally, I've learned a small meditation technique that only takes minutes, but will help you tune into what your body is feeling. You only need a chair and a few minutes. You can even do it in your car while sitting at a park or while sitting on a couch in a client's home.

Sit with your feet on the ground and your hands on your thighs. Your eyes don't have to be shut but relax your lids. Relax your jaw and put your tongue just behind your front teeth. Roll your shoulders, and then drop them. Take a big breath, hold for two counts, then release. Begin your check-in. Start with the top of your head. How does it feel? Move to your ears. Focus on the sensation of your ears. Do they hurt? Are they ringing? Just make a note of it. Move onto your eyes, your nose and your mouth. Check in with your jaw. Does it hurt from grinding your teeth? Did you know that you grind your teeth? Make a mental note and move on.

Check in with your shoulders. Be sure they are relaxed and dropped. Check in with your arms. How do they feel? If they are tense, relax them. Check in with your hands. They should be heavy and warm on your thighs. Next, check in with your chest. Breathe in and breathe out. Check in with your abdomen. Pain? Where? Make a mental note of it. Continue checking in with your hips and lower back.

Then check your thighs and knees. Are they relaxed? Check in with your shins and your calves. Relax them. Lastly, check in with your feet. Are they aching? Make a mental note. Once you've completed checking in, take a deep breath and let it out. Now take those mental notes and write them down. These are things you may need to visit your doctor about, learn to relax into or address in another way such as massage or stretches.

This body check in can take as long as you want it to, but usually takes me about 10 minutes. However, if you find you only have two minutes, you can still do a quick version. The point is to stop what you're doing and check in with yourself.

*If you find that your negative self-talk is also including self-harm or thoughts of suicide do not hesitate to call for help: **1-800-273-TALK** (8255).

Friends & Family - Work on developing and improving relationships with your friends and family. If you are suffering from compassion fatigue, chances are you've already isolated yourself and shut them out. It is important to reach out to one of your most trusted family members or friends and let them into your sphere. It's going to be difficult, but the support and love you receive will encourage you to let others in to help you. A supportive circle of friends and family will help you along the recovery process. Let them know you are struggling with compassion fatigue.

If they don't know what it is, I've listed a few resources at the end of this book that you can research together for a better understanding of your situation. Let them listen to you. If you find that they are troubled by your stories, then seek the help of a professional who may not be traumatized by your stories. If you have a church family, you could ask them to pray for you without giving details. If you have a network of professional colleagues, you could ask them to study compassion fatigue as a group. If you have a Facebook friend who you seem to connect with, you can ask them to be an accountability partner to keep your self-talk in a positive tone.

Be creative, be open, but please let someone in. Cultivating relationships while battling compassion fatigue may seem impossible. You may be thinking you would only bring them down or ruin their fun. Let them be the judge of that. You only need to reach out. Take small steps. Go for a short walk with a friend. Go have a cup of coffee with a peer. Small steps will lead to a sense of self-awareness and mindfulness. I'd recommend that you check in with your friends and family in person, rather than a text or a Facebook message. I know it's exhausting to have to get out of your PJs, brush your hair and get dressed, but the effort is worth it. You don't have to be an overachiever with this step either. Once a week to begin with is great!

Keep in mind that compassion fatigue concerning pet sitters has not been studied by scientists yet. We straddle two worlds; the world of caring for pets and the world of caring for people. Because we are in client's homes, we are also privy to things that the rest of the world isn't. Until the world of science catches up with our industry and begins to study our world and the effects of trauma and moral distress, we must find our healing in the worlds that have already been studied and explored: human caregivers and animal caregivers in shelters and veterinary clinics. Some of the ideas and suggestions will apply to us. Some will not. Take what you need and leave the rest. Be assured that science will catch up to us and there are a few scientists who already know that we are suffering. You are not alone.

Hope

I knew I was beginning to heal when I started to seek out other people's dogs to pet them. I was burning to know: What's the dog's name? How old is he/she? What breed is she/he? The rush of emotion I used to feel when I'd put my hands in the ruff of a dog's neck started to come back. It was small at first, a twinkle not a spark.

One day, my husband and I were on the beach at Puget Sound. We met a young man there collecting driftwood that the Pacific Ocean had deposited. This young strong man was hauling the logs by hand into his truck. He was using the wood to create art. He was passionate about his art. He had returned from the Iraq, the Sand Box as he called it, only a few years before and the art was his way of dealing with his own case of PTSD.

As we spoke, I felt a poke in my thigh. Looking down, I met the gaze of an enormous pit bill with a mischievous grin and a very big stick. He poked me, again. I realized he wanted to play and as I knelt down to pet him, he poked me again. His dad just laughed and said, "He wants you to throw it." So, I obliged him. I thought I'd have to wrestle the stick out of his mouth, but he promptly dropped it at my feet. I chucked that stick into the water with all of my might. The dog gave me a glance as if to say, "That's it?" and plunged into the water after his stick, which actually was a small log.

It didn't take the dog long to figure out that I couldn't throw the stick as far as his dad and he lowered his expectations of me. He came splashing back to me, put his stick at my feet and the shook the sea water off of his coat and all over my jeans. Then, he waited for my reaction. I looked him right in the eye, bent over and picked up his stick. This action sent the dog into a place of sheer bliss and he let out a happy bark. I threw the stick again, and he went plunging back into the Sound to retrieve his stick.

Shocked, I realized dogs hadn't been drawn to me as they had been before. I think they must have somehow known that I needed time and space. But that day, that silly pit bull poked my thigh with that stick and I threw it for him over and over again, laughing with him until my belly hurt. It felt like a ray of light breaking through dense storm clouds.

Since that day, I have been paying attention to dogs' behavior around me, and to my delight, they are seeking me out again. I also realized that I am willing to stop what I am doing to meet a new dog, an action I had stopped doing when compassion fatigue set in.

My sparkle was coming back. Putting my pants on became a little easier. I started to joke with my husband and make him laugh again. I started to tease my son with ridiculous puns that he says he hates, but always make him smile. I know I've hit the mark with him when he says, "just stop!" and dramatically walks away from me. He always comes back and hugs me though. I started humming again too. Unbeknownst to me, I hum when I'm content. My son noticed it first and mentioned he hadn't heard me hum in several years. I hadn't noticed until he mentioned it.

I also noticed that I could walk my own dogs without the graphic intrusive images and the intolerance to loud noises and strong smells. I started to enjoy my new environment. My anxiety was starting to wane and I was sleeping better. Knowing we'd soon be away from the bully also filled me with the hope that my recovery would accelerate.

Then came a gift wrapped in a fur coat. I was given an opportunity to see how much compassion had actually been renewed and how resilient I actually am. A dog had been abandoned in a car in the parking lot of our condo complex.

It was a complicated story, but basically, the owner of the dog had been arrested, leaving the dog in the car with the windows rolled down. It was winter and, in Seattle, it rains every day. With the windows down, the dog and the car were very wet. I found out about this dog 24 hours after her dad had been arrested. Our whole community was buzzing about it, yet not one person did anything about it. Many postings of outrage and concern appeared on our community website, but no one stepped up to actually help the dog.

I called the Sheriff and Animal Control to get advice and then made the decision to get the dog out of the car for a walk and some food. There were conflicting rules and laws involved between the Sheriff and Animal Control. I tried not to break the rules, but the care of the dog came first and I really didn't care who was going to tell me differently. It turns out there is a Good Samaritan Law in Washington that covered me for the first 72 hours I was involved with the dog. Tony supported me 100%, even if I was breaking a rule or two.

I visited her multiple times over the course of four days, feeding her, giving her water and walking her. It was soon uncovered that her dad had *borrowed* the car from his roommate, who didn't even know it was missing. Deputies got in touch with him so he could retrieve the car and the dog. The dog, who I named Jane, needed help and no one was willing to step up, despite their huffing and puffing about it. So I did.

Quietly, with only the authorities and Tony knowing what I was doing, I cared for and comforted Jane. I told her what a lovely sparkly collar she had and reassured her that someone must love her to buy her such a dazzling collar. I realized, as my heart filled with emotion for Jane, that she must be lonely and confused. My compassion was reigniting. A year earlier, I would have let this slide and the dog would have suffered. It would have been someone else's responsibility to call the authorities and I would have left it up to someone else to take care of her. But when this situation presented itself, I didn't hesitate.

The instinct to care for her rose in me and I followed it. There was much talk about how cruel her dad was for leaving her, how angry people were at the authorities for not taking her to the shelter and what an unsightly mess this was in our parking lot. People talk. I respect the ones who take action like the Sheriff and the Animal Control Officer who helped me care for Jane.

I can say, without any doubt in my mind, that Jane was an answer for me. I met her for a reason. I had to go through this situation with Jane to see that my compassion was still there bubbling up through the anxiety.

Dogs teach us things if we only listen. When this ordeal was over, my husband said to me, while I was sitting among notes and messages from all the phone calls and emails thanking me for my actions, "Now THAT'S what Holly does!"

I have since taken my education about compassion fatigue to heart and committed to share what I have learned with other pet sitters who may be suffering. I am sharing my story in the hopes that others can start their own recovery process. It is why I wrote this book and why I am making presentations on this topic at conferences and meetings for those in the pet care industry.

I also maintain a blog (hollyccook.com) to share my own experiences and lessons. I have written this book and am working on a companion guide to recovery from Compassion Fatigue, and co-writing a research paper on the subject while continuing to run my business. I continue to walk dogs in Seattle but have decided to stop pet sitting. I've also become a certified Compassion Fatigue Educator through The University of Tennessee School of Social Work. We cannot address this issue until we all acknowledge this is a rampant problem in our industry. I know it is and I know there is help.

My life has changed immeasurably in the last few years and all for the better. There is hope and, if you are suffering, you are not alone. My wish is that this book will bring you hope, relief and permission to begin your journey into healing. There is a ray of light peeking through the storm clouds of your pain. Let it shine and each of you can recover your sparkle, too.

Acknowledgements

I am grateful for the support of loved ones and friends who encouraged me to tell my story in the hopes that it will help others suffering from Compassion Fatigue. If I were to acknowledge each and every person and pet who helped me along my journey, this book would be another 50 pages long.

If you are reading this book, let me say thank you for reading the acknowledgments and taking a peek into my life. My wish is that this book will bring you hope, relief and permission to begin your journey into healing. There is a ray of light peeking through the storm clouds of your pain. Let it shine.

My sincere thanks to anyone in the pet care industry, including pet sitters, dog walkers, veterinarians, vet techs, animal shelter workers and, especially, those who respond to a pet in need. We are kindred spirits and I understand what compels you.

My gratitude should begin with my parents, of course, for allowing me to follow my passion for animals and never turning me away when I had an animal in distress in my arms.

My gratitude and abounding love to Tony, my steadfast helpmate, always at my side through thick and thin, who supports me no matter what kind of shenanigans I get myself into. Sometimes my heart is so full of love for you that I am rendered speechless. Thank you for being my husband.

My gratitude and unconditional love to my son, Cyle, who loves to challenge me and who surpasses my expectations every day. His support and constant reminders to be true to myself got me through many challenges. I'm proud to be his Mum.

My love and gratitude to all of the dogs in my personal life; Bruno, Rusty, Pansy, Petunia, Tulip, Toots, Boots, Weasel, Wooley Bear, Bear, Glace Mae, Rufus, Sarah (who chewed up my wedding gown), Sam, Hazel, and Mozi. Each one of these dogs taught me about unconditional love.

My unending gratitude to every single client and pet of Special Pet Care Services, LLC, and Northwest Dog Walking Company both in Michigan and Seattle. My days were filled in the company of many special pets and I want to list every single one of them right here, for each one of them taught me something of value. They were all my best friends. And Slider, the hero Greyhound, who took a bite in the shoulder from a charging German Shepherd so it wouldn't bite me. He saved me.

A very special thanks to Mary, Samantha, LuAnn, Diane, Laurie, Kelli, Brenna and their families for working with me and sharing your family members.

You are all extraordinary pet sitters and I'm proud of you.

A special thanks to Cathy Vaughn and Michelle Romano for being brave enough to allow me to speak about Compassion Fatigue during the first ever Texas Pet Sitter's Convention in San Antonio in 2016. Compassion Fatigue is an epidemic in the animal care industry, and these two ladies were brave enough to encourage me to tell my story for the first time.

Huge thanks to all the attendees of the first ever Texas Pet Sitter's Convention for they were all so supportive of my story; especially Lorena. She knows why.

Thank you to Donna Fuller, who wrote Happy Work, Happy Life; An Inside Job, who I met at the aforementioned conference. We are cut from the same cloth and I am grateful for your support and help getting this book written.

Thank you to Melissa Roth for taking on this project and bringing my words to life. Thank you for your constant support and encouraging words. Thank you for your hard work and long hours. I'm sure it wasn't easy reading this over and over and over again.

A special thanks to Cindy Vet and Josh Cary for believing in the power of my story. Thank you for another opportunity to tell my story at PSO 2016 and for pushing me to share my story. I'm still not sure about it, but I'm confident you guys know what you are talking about, so I persevere.

Thank you to the authors of my favorite books; Dr. Sophia Yin, Dr. Marty Becker, James Herriot, Jon Katz, W. Bruce Cameron, M. Scott Peck M.D., Suzanne Clothier and, believe it or not, Trixie Koontz, Dean Koontz's Golden Retriever. Each of these authors has had an impact in my life.

Additionally, I'd like to thank the scientists and researchers who study Compassion Fatigue and the authors of books and papers that helped me write this book; Dr. Susan Cohen, Dr. Charles Figley, Dr. Bernard Rollin Ph.D., Francois Mathieu, Debbie L. Stoewen, DVM, MSW, RSW, Ph.D. and many others.

Finally, thank you to Jessica Dolce, for building her Compassion In Balance course and for educating the world about Compassion Fatigue. Jessica, you are literally saving lives.

Recommended Research:

1. Any book about Compassion Fatigue by Dr. Charles Figley.
2. Trauma Stewardship Laura van Dernoot Kipsky
3. Sign up for Compassion In Balance with Jessica Dolce. Online course. www.jessicadolce.com

About the Author

*Wife of Tony
*Mum to Cyle
*Pet Parent to Hazel, Mozi, Chrissy & Polly
*Certified Compassion Fatigue Instructor (University of Tennessee School Of Social Work)
*Certified K9 Obedience Trainer (Specializing in puppies)
*Award Winning Pet Sitter Extraordinaire (Over 20 years serving my community and their pets)
*Walker of Dogs, large or small, shy or friendly, comical or stoic, athletic or lazy. I love them all.
*Caregiver to Cats, whom are usually not impressed by accolades.
*Compassionate advocate for pets and their parents facing end of life decisions. (That's a tough gig)
*Enthusiastic educator of the public about pet sitting and the pet sitting industry
*Superhero for pets in disasters
*Crazy dog lady that organizes community service events for my town

If you ventured this far into my book, then your curiosity has gotten the best of you and I will respect your query. I started pet sitting in 1994, winning Pet Sitter of the Year in 2004; an award given by Pet Sitters International

I have served my industry by becoming a state Ambassador for PSI in 2005. I have authored several articles about pet sitting and have presented at several   conferences. I have served my community with a yearly Christmas donation drive for local shelters. I also served to educate local community services about pet sitting and pet care. Additionally, I developed several programs through my business that focused on community service. I have developed donation drives for communities devastated by disaster (From Missouri floods in 1993, 9/11, Hurricane Katrina to Hurricane Sandy.)

I am currently compelled to reach out to the pet sitting industry to educate about Compassion Fatigue. Why would I do that? Because I have fought that demon and there were scarce resources to assist me. I am determined to help pet sitters specifically, who are suffering from Compassion Fatigue.

Please follow my blog at hollyccook.com.

Watch for my Compassion Fatigue In Pet Sitting Workbook coming in the Spring 2017.

www.ingramcontent.com/pod-product-compliance
Lightning Source LLC
Chambersburg PA
CBHW020535290526
45786CB00002B/891